LIVE
Your Life
WITH
COPD

52 WEEKS OF
Health, Happiness, and Hope

SECOND EDITION

JANE M. MARTIN, BA, CRT
based on the editorials of Jo-Von Tucker

outskirts
press

Dedication

*This book is dedicated to the people with chronic
obstructive pulmonary disease (COPD).
You humble me. You honor me. You are
my teachers and my inspiration.*

Table of Contents – Calendar Method

Dedication

What People Are Saying About Live Your Life with COPD I

Medical Disclaimer III

Acknowledgments IV

Introduction – A Story of Two Women V

How to Get the Most out of This Book IX

About COPD XII

Foreword IV

A Word from the Author XV

January Week 1 – Happy New Year!   JVT 1

January Week 2 – Know Your Numbers –
   Pulmonary Function Testing   JMM 4

Added Insight -- How to ask for spirometry –
   a question for Helen Sorenson 6

January Week 3 – Your Relationship
   with Your Doctor JVT/JMM... 8

January Week 4 – Defying the Laws of
   Gravity…or…Holding on to Stability   JVT............................. 12

January Week 5 – Reclaiming Your Life
   through Pulmonary Rehabilitation   JMM.............................. 17

Added Insight – Nick's story... 21

February Week 1 – Your Relationship with Others and
the Need to Love, and Be Loved   JVT/JMM 25
February Week 2 – COPD Research   JMM 31
February Week 3 – Good Days, Bad Days   JVT 36
Added Insight I – How the weather affects breathing 38
Added Insight II – Morning body scan, Mindful meditation.......... 39
February Week 4 – Panic and Anxiety in COPD   VS................... 42

March Week 1 – Panic Attack! The Anatomy and
Physiology of a Panic Attack   VS 47
Added Insight – How can I tell if it's panic? –
a question for Dr. Sharma .... .51
March Week 2 – Accentuate the Positive –
Every Day is a Gift JVT... 55
March Week 3 – Travel with COPD and Oxygen   JVT/JMM 60
March Week 4 – A Look at the Lungs –
How are They Supposed to Work and
What Went Wrong?   JMM 65
Added Insight – Oxygen transport and
obstructive vs. restrictive lung disease.................................... 72
March Week 5 – Compassion, Renewal,
and Rediscovery with COPD   JVT... .75

April Week 1 – Could You Have Alpha-1?   JMM......................... 79
Added Insight – John Walsh's story 83
April Week 2 – How to be Able-Hearted
When You Can't be Able-Bodied   JVT/JMM 87
Added Insight – Jeanette's story... 90
April Week 3 – Nutrition   JMM 93
April Week 4 – Coping with Stress   JVT 102

May Week 1 – The Emotional Impact of
　　Being Diagnosed and Living with COPD　JMM 106
Added Insight – Helping ourselves –
　　a question for Dr. Sharma 110
May Week 2 – Making the Most of the
　　Breath You Have – Energy Conservation
　　and Work Simplification　JMM 112
Added Insight I – Climbing stairs 116
Added Insight II – In the kitchen 117
May Week 3 – Gardening and Yardwork　JMM 120
May Week 4 – Exercise　JMM 126
Added Insight – Should I exercise when I'm sick?
　　– a question for Helen Sorenson 129

June Week 1 – What Can I Count on Today?　JMM/JVT 132
June Week 2 – Dying with COPD　JMM 137
Added Insight – Dale's story 141
June Week 3 – Your Questions about Oxygen
　　with Answers from Lung Professionals　FA/RS/HS 145
June Week 4 – COPD: Unseen
　　and Misunderstood　JVT/JMM 151

July Week 1 – Learning to Breathe Again –
　　Part I: Pursed-Lips Breathing　JMM 154
July Week 2 – Learning to Breathe Again –
　　Part II: Diaphragmatic Breathing　JMM 160
Added Insight – A tip on practicing
　　diaphragmatic breathing from Helen Sorenson 164
July Week 3 – Relaxation　VS 166
July Week 4 – Keeping a Journal　JVT 174
Added Insight – Bonnie's story 176
July Week 5 – Medications　JMM 178
Added Insight – Melissa's story 187

August Week 1 – Hope   JVT 192

Added Insight – Steve's thoughts on hope 194

August Week 2 – Worry   VS 197

August Week 3 – Stages of COPD: Where Am I
    and What Does it Mean?   JMM 203

August Week 4 – Making the Most of Living
    with Advanced COPD   JMM 209

September Week 1 – Harmonica Playing with COPD   JMM...... 214

September Week 2 – Have I Got a Cure for You!
    Understanding Alternative Treatments for COPD   RS 221

Added Insight – Stem cell therapy... 226

September Week 3 – Facing Fall – Preventing
    Exacerbations and When to Call the Doctor   JMM 230

September Week 4 – Cough and Airway Clearance   JMM 236

Added Insight – When Coughing is too Distasteful –
    An article by Dr. Adams.. 240

September Week 5 – Denial   JMM.. 245

Added Insight I – Tom's Story 251

Added Insight II – Eileen's Story 252

October Week 1 – Advance Directives – Why You
    (and everybody) Should Have a Living Will   JMM 256

October Week 2 – Depression   JMM 261

October Week 3 – Additional Therapies for COPD:
    Massage, Yoga, Tai chi, and Qigong JMM............................ 266

Added Insight – Debbie's Story 269

October Week 4 – Losing Someone with COPD   JVT/JMM 272

Added Insight – Do Not Stand at My Grave and Weep 27

November Week 1 – Isolation with COPD
and Why we Need Emotional Support   JVT 277
November Week 2 – Ten Tips to Enjoy the Holidays   JMM 281
November Week 3 – A Time of Thanksgiving   JVT 285
Added Insight – John's thoughts on being thankful 287
November Week 4 – Dear Family and
Friends, in a Perfect World…   JVT 291

December Week 1 – War or Peace?   JVT/JMM 297
Added Insight – Quitting Smoking – Letters of support
from Betty, Linda, Kay, Arlene, and John 300
December Week 2 – Party Time! Nine Tips
to Help you Save Energy and Breathe Better
This Holiday Season   JMM 304
December Week 3 – A COPD Christmas   Jim Phillips 308
December Week 4 – Thoughts About the Future   JVT 311

Authors' and Contributors' Biographies 314
Glossary 320
Resources 328

Table of Contents: Content Method

To find the page number of the chapter you're looking for, and for the complete Table of Contents, see the Table of Contents – Calendar Method.

The Basics

January Week 2 – Know Your Numbers – Pulmonary Function Testing
Added Insight – How to ask for spirometry –
    a question for Helen Sorenson
January Week 5 – Reclaiming Your
    Life Through Pulmonary Rehabilitation
Added Insight – Nick's story
February Week 2 – COPD Research
March Week 3 – Travel with COPD and Oxygen
March Week 4 – A Look at the Lungs –
    How are They Supposed to Work and What Went Wrong?
Added Insight – Oxygen transport and
    restrictive vs. obstructive lung disease
April Week 1 – Could You Have Alpha-1?
Added Insight – John Walsh's story
April Week 3 – Nutrition
May Week 2 – Making the Most of the Breath You Have –
    Energy Conservation and Work Simplification
Added Insight I – Climbing stairs
Added Insight II – In the kitchen
May Week 4 – Exercise
Added Insight – Should I exercise when I'm sick? –
    a question for Helen Sorenson
June Week 3 – Your Questions About Oxygen

with Answers from Lung Professionals

July Week 1 – Learning to Breathe Again –
    Part I: Pursed-Lips Breathing

July Week 2 – Learning to Breathe Again –
    Part II: Diaphragmatic Breathing

Added Insight – A tip on practicing
    diaphragmatic breathing from Helen Sorenson

July Week 3 – Relaxation

July Week 5 – Medications

Added Insight – Melissa's Story

August Week 3 – Stages of COPD: Where Am
    I and What Does it Mean?

September Week 2 – Have I Got a Cure for You!
    Understanding Alternative Treatments for COPD

Added Insight – Stem cell therapy

September Week 3 – Facing Fall –
    Preventing Exacerbations and When to Call the Doctor

September Week 4 – Cough and Airway Clearance

Added Insight – When Coughing is too Distasteful –
    an article by Dr. Adams

October Week 3 – Additional Therapies for COPD:
    Massage, Yoga, Tai chi, and Qigong

Added Insight – Debbie's Story

Relationships

January Week 3 – Your Relationship with Your Doctor

February Week 1 – Your Relationship with Others and
    the Need to Love, and Be Loved

November Week 1 – Isolation with COPD
    and Why we Need Emotional Support

November Week 4 – Dear Family and Friends, in a Perfect World…

Day-to-Day Living

January Week 4 – Defying the Laws of Gravity…
    or…Holding on to Stability
February Week 3 – Good Days, Bad Days
Added Insight I – How the weather affects breathing
Added Insight II – Morning body scan, Mindful meditation
April Week 2 – How to be Able-Hearted
    When You Can't be Able-Bodied
Added Insight – Jeanette's story
May Week 3 – Gardening and Yardwork
June Week 1 – What Can I Count on Today?
June Week 4 – COPD: Unseen and Misunderstood
July Week 4 – Keeping a Journal
Added Insight – Bonnie's story
August Week 4 – Making the Most of Living
    with Advanced COPD
September Week 1 – Harmonica Playing with COPD
November Week 2 – Ten Tips to Enjoy the Holidays
November Week 3 – A Time of Thanksgiving
Added Insight – John's thoughts on being thankful
December Week 2 – Party Time! Nine Tips to Help
    You Save Energy and Breathe Better This Holiday Season

Emotional Issues and Coping

January Week 1 – Happy New Year!
February Week 4 – Panic and Anxiety in COPD
March Week 1 – Panic Attack! The Anatomy
    and Physiology of a Panic Attack
Added Insight – How can I tell if it's panic? – a question for Dr. Sharma
March Week 2 – Accentuate the Positive – Every Day is a Gift
March Week 5 – Compassion, Renewal, and Rediscovery with COPD

April Week 4 – Coping with Stress
May Week 1 – The Emotional Impact of Being
    Diagnosed and Living With COPD
Added Insight – Helping Ourselves – a question for Dr. Sharma
August Week 1 – Hope
Added Insight – Steve's thoughts on hope
August Week 2 – Worry
September Week 5 – Denial
Added Insight I – Tom's Story
Added Insight II – Eileen's Story
October Week 2 – Depression
December Week 1 – War or Peace?
Added Insight – Quitting Smoking – Letters of support
    from Betty, Linda, Kay, Arlene, and John
December Week 4 – Thoughts About the Future

Living and Dying with COPD

June Week 2 – Dying with COPD
Added Insight – Dale's story
October Week 1 – Advance Directives –
    Why You (and everybody) Should Have a Living Will
October Week 4 – Losing Someone with COPD
Added Insight – Do not Stand at My Grave and Weep

Just for Fun

December Week 3 – A COPD Christmas

What people are saying about Live Your Life with COPD - 52 Weeks of Health, Happiness, and Hope

Second edition

Live Your Life with COPD - 52 Weeks of Health, Happiness, and Hope is a guide for living with COPD, an important issue that affects so many. It has information and education throughout as well as inspiring stories; yet, it is a fresh read, easy to follow, and hard to put down. What really stood out to me were the main points to remember at the end of the week and suggestions on things to try.

Marshall Swanson, COPD patient

Jane's book provides detailed information from beginning to end about COPD and outlines how to live with COPD from the first time one is diagnosed. This book kept me wanting to learn more about how to manage my disease. Thank you, Jane for helping us continue to find our way through this journey of ups, downs, and unknowns. Your book is a blueprint for us to follow as we go through the hills and valleys of this disease.

Janice Cotton, COPD patient and advocate

Having COPD isn't a choice, but how one lives with it is. I could sit on the couch with a hose in my nose, but I know that is a slippery slope and hard to climb back from. So, I choose to LIVE my life and stay active and enjoy each day. You can do that too. Live Your Life with COPD - 52 Weeks of Health, Happiness, and Hope shows you how.
John Linnell, Living with COPD and COPD Advocate

This book will help tremendously for life with COPD, through struggles with depression and learning to cope and live with COPD, as well as with comorbidities that are associated with COPD. It will give Courage, Hope, Encouragement, and Happiness to maintain health, and the strength to maintain quality of life. The reality is that I have COPD, but it does not have me.
Tina Moyer, COPD patient and advocate

Live Your Life with COPD - 52 Weeks of Health, Happiness, and Hope is a beautiful, bountiful "basket" of comprehensive COPD self-care. If I had to carry just one book with me, this would be it. Thank you for putting in the yeoman's effort in composing this work. It will undoubtedly be of great help to the newly diagnosed as well as long-diagnosed people with COPD.
Peg Johnson, COPD patient

Medical Disclaimer

This book is not intended as medical advice or to take the place of an authorized medical professional. You, the reader, are encouraged to discuss the information in this book with your doctor or other qualified healthcare professional. Together you can determine the best treatment and care for your individual situation.

Acknowledgments

I am grateful to Jo-Von Tucker who not only wrote about the physical, social, and emotional challenges in life with COPD, but moreover, had the courage to put it out there. Her spirit lives on in this book.

Thank you to Dr. Frank Adams, Dr. Robert "Sandy" Sandhaus, Dr. Vijai Sharma, and Helen Sorenson, RRT for their professional contributions to the first edition and their review of the second. Many thanks to Dr. Barbara Yawn, Professor of Family and Community Health at the University of Minnesota for reviewing select chapters.

I am grateful to Debbie Daro for telling us about her experience with Tai chi and Qigong; and to Stacey Blank, Darcy Ellefson, and Dave P. Folds III, for sharing their stories about starting and maintaining their harmonica programs.

My thanks goes to LinDee Rochelle for her professionalism as my editor and her empathy as a fellow author; and to Shannon Finney for patiently providing the interior artwork. I thank my fellow authors who, by their friendship and example, encourage me to march on and get the job done.

My deep appreciation is owed to the true experts, those with COPD, for sharing their stories and cheering me on. You are the reason I love what I do. You teach me and inspire me.

Finally, I thank my husband, Marvin, for taking care of a thousand everyday things with never a complaint, and for giving me the time and space to write and be me.

Introduction – A Story of Two Women

I didn't choose to write this book. It chose me.

When I was doing research for my first book, I heard about a new book about COPD written by a patient, a lady named Jo-Von Tucker. As I read it, I was struck by Jo-Von's honesty in telling what it was like to fight the day-to-day battle for health and breath. The emotional issues in life with COPD can be brutal. Jo-Von courageously shared herself with readers, revealing her fears, her demons, her failings, her triumphs, her hopes.

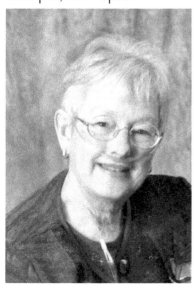

Jo-Von Tucker

She wrote about the very issues – the emotional struggles – I'd seen in my own patients. On the road they traveled, sometimes my patients would stumble and fall, at times it was as if they were swallowed by a sinkhole. More often than not, though, they'd pick themselves up and march on, even stronger than before. But every time, every single time – by just being assured they were not alone – they were inspired.

I, myself, don't have COPD, but from my experience as a respiratory therapist, I knew then, more than anything, that this information – this side of life with COPD – must come to light. That's why I wrote my first book; so folks with COPD who were doing well, those who'd faced the issues and conquered them, could help others.

I was in awe of Jo-Von, who had not only beat the odds to live on and live well with COPD but had written a comprehensive guide to doing just that. After all, she was a successful businesswoman, who, at age fifty-two was diagnosed with COPD and told she had only two to five years to live. Undaunted, she went on to become a well-known advocate for people with COPD and a support group leader, speaker and writer.

With a leap of faith, I contacted Jo-Von through email, not sure if she'd open it in the first place, give me another thought if she did, let alone write back. But she did. We soon became friends and sup-ported each other in both our writing and in the often-challenging process of publishing. Others wrote about things like medications and nutrition for COPD; yes, we were writing about that, but so much more. We wrote with care and sensitivity what was in the hearts and minds of people with COPD. Jo-Von and I were kindred spirits in that regard, pretty much the only ones at that time writing about the emo-tional issues associated with COPD.

Jo-Von put me on the mailing list for her Cape Cod Support Group newsletter. I looked forward each month to reading about events and concerns from her group because I, too, ran a support group in my hometown. But without a doubt, the first piece I'd look for was her editorial. So often I'd think, "Boy, she hit the nail on the head with this one! Real people feel this way, but they just don't talk about it. And here she is, putting it down on paper."

Our friendship grew. Jo-Von introduced me by phone to a col-league of hers, Dr. Austin "Bill" Kutscher who organized COPD symposiums in New York City. In November of 2003 I finally met both Jo-Von and Bill in person at the first national COPD Coalition meeting in Arlington, Virginia. I found Jo-Von at her presentation in the poster room. I met Bill later that night. He was a wiry man with a slight build, in his eighties, with a ferocious energy and intensity.

Barely a month later I was shocked and saddened to learn that Jo-Von passed away unexpectedly from complications following surgery. In corresponding with her over three years through email, I'd always looked forward to meeting her someday, which thankfully I did, and working with her. That latter hope, of course, was now gone. Or, was it?

The following June Bill invited me to speak at a COPD symposium at Columbia University Medical Center in New York City. He asked that I present two papers; one I'd written, and the other written by Jo-Von that she had planned to present. At the close of the first day of the event, Bill handed me a stack of papers held together by a rubber band.

"Jane, these are Jo-Von's editorials. You should have them."

"Um…okay… thank you," I answered, not really understanding what he meant by giving them to me, nor knowing what he wanted me to do with them.

That night in my hotel room, I re-read the newsletters, one after the other, spreading them out on my bed, overcome again by the wisdom in those forty-some editorials within 150 pages of her writings. It was a joy to see Jo-Von's words, the entire collection here in front of me; open, positive, hopeful words of a wise woman with COPD. With a renewed sense of purpose, I read of her experiences, her insights, her wisdom, her questions, as she shared her mind and heart and spirit … all with her own brand of gusto and that no-nonsense Texas/Manhattan style. I knew that night – somehow this work had to be shared so Jo-Von's legacy could live on.

The next day I said to Bill, "I read the editorials."

His eyes met mine. "Yes?"

I thought, *Jane, you've got an awful lot of nerve, but you have to say what you believe*. I came right out with it. "They should be in a book."

He smiled. "I was hoping you'd say that. And you're the one to do it."

Stunned first, by Bill's trust in me, a moment later, I realized the weight of this responsibility. Six years later I finished the book. I regret never having the pleasure to work with my friend Jo-Von directly, but in working with her editorials, in way, I did. It was a joy and an honor as much now as it was then. I'm delighted to share with you this second edition of *Live Your Life with COPD - 52 Weeks of Health, Happiness, and Hope*.

Jane Martin's first book was *Breathe Better, Live in Wellness: Winning Your Battle over Shortness of Breath*. Jo-Von's book is *Courage and Inspiration for Life with Chronic Obstructive Pulmonary Disease*.

How to Get the Most Out of This Book

Live Your Life with COPD - 52 Weeks of Health, Happiness and Hope is organized as a perpetual calendar with 52 chapters, one for each week of the year. Some chapters focus on seasonal events or specific issues relevant to that time of year.

People with COPD often feel overwhelmed with all there is to learn about managing this disease, not to mention the wide array of emotional issues. Dedicating one chapter per week to each topic is designed to give you, the reader, time to focus, learn, and use what you find in each chapter.

But as solid as this information may be, reading is still passive. This is why at the end of each chapter you'll find "Your Turn," which includes key points, thoughtful questions, suggested tasks, and goals. You're encouraged to think about how the topic relates to you and put possible solutions into practice. At the end of some chapters an "Added Insight" offers additional information or inspiration.

By all means, if this is your copy of *Live Your Life with COPD*, I encourage you to jot notes and thoughts in the book itself. If you've borrowed this copy from a friend or the library, keep a notebook with it so you, too, can fully participate in "Your Turn."

There are three options for how to use this book.

1.) Calendar Method

Let's say you're ready to start reading and it happens to be the fourth week in April. In that case you would start with the chapter "April – Week 4: Coping with Stress." From there you can go right through to the end of the book, then continue on with "January – Week 1" until you finish with "April – Week 3: Nutrition."

2.) Content Method

If you prefer learning first about the basics of living with COPD, such as lung function, medications, nutrition, exercise, etc., see the other table of contents – Content Method. Here, chapters are organized by categories and topics.

3.) Browsing Method

You may want to skip around to chapters that interest you at the moment. If you choose to do this, however, put a checkmark in the table of contents for chapters you've covered. 52 chapters is a lot to keep track of and I wouldn't want you to miss anything!

Credits

This book is based on, and inspired by, the editorials of the late Jo-Von Tucker. Some chapters are essentially unchanged from the original editorials. These chapters are credited as JVT. (Author initials can be found in the Table of Contents - Calendar Method.)

Some chapters originating from Jo-Von's editorials have been updated and/or more significantly edited. In doing so, I've done my best to be true to her message and her voice. These chapters are credited

JVT/JMM.

Chapters authored by me are based on years of teaching people with COPD and other lung diseases and are credited as JMM. I knew I was on the right track when individuals in a pulmonary rehabilitation class or breathing support group audience nodded as I spoke. Later they would come up to me and say, "Thank you. This makes sense to me now. I finally understand it."

At the beginning of chapters authored, or contributed, by our expert contributors: Dr. Frank Adams, Dr. Robert Sandhaus, Dr. Vijai Sharma, and respiratory therapist Helen Sorenson, you will find their initials. (See authors' and contributors' biographies at the end of this book.)

Welcome to Live Your Life with COPD - 52 Weeks of Health, Happiness, and Hope, your guide to living well with chronic obstructive pulmonary disease. I wish for you the discovery of solid information, thoughtful perspectives, joyful inspiration, and endless empowerment. Whether you were diagnosed ten years ago, or just yesterday, come along with us now on this journey, a journey of not just weeks – but years – of *Health, Happiness, and Hope.*

About COPD

What is COPD?

Chronic obstructive pulmonary disease (COPD) is a term used to describe chronic lung diseases including emphysema and chronic bronchitis. This disease is characterized by increasing breathlessness.

Although COPD is a progressive and currently incurable disease, with the right diagnosis and treatment, individuals can manage their COPD and breathe better. People can live for many years with COPD and enjoy life.

What are the symptoms?

COPD can be different for each person, but common symptoms are:

- Increased shortness of breath
- Frequent coughing (with and without mucus)
- Increased breathlessness
- Wheezing
- Tightness in the chest

What causes COPD?

Most often COPD is caused by inhaling pollutants. The most

common is tobacco smoke from cigarettes, pipes, cigars, etc. COPD is caused also by second-hand smoke, as well as fumes, chemicals, and dust found in many work environments. Smoke and fumes from some cooking fuels in the home can also be contributing factors in the development of COPD.

Genetics can play a role. Alpha-1 Antitrypsin Deficiency is a genetically inherited disorder that can lead to COPD and/or liver disease. In Alpha-1 even those who have never smoked or have never been exposed to strong lung irritants in their environment, can develop COPD at a young age.

How common is COPD and what is its impact?

- Nearly 16 million adults have COPD and millions more are undiagnosed or developing COPD.
- COPD is the fourth leading cause of death in the US, killing more than 150,000 people each year.
- Despite the high number of deaths, COPD ranks 155th in research funding from the National Institutes of Health (NIH).
- COPD kills more women than men each year, nearly twice as many as breast cancer.
- The World Health Organization (WHO) estimates that more than 250 million individuals worldwide have COPD.
- Most people are not diagnosed with COPD until they have lost half of their lung function.

Source: COPD Foundation   www.copfoundation.org

Foreword

I've known Jane Martin for many years, and I've always appreciated her contributions to support and educate those with COPD. As we are both respiratory therapists, patient advocates, and writers, we share a mutual respect. And yes, we've shared some fun times as well, in long talks at professional conferences and in preparation for Jane serving as guest speaker on a Sea Puffer Cruise. I also knew Jo-Von Tucker. She, too, was a kindred spirit in the work of writing and advocating for those with COPD.

In this book Jane takes her many years of experience working in acute care, leading breathing support groups, coordinating pulmonary rehabilitation, and working with the COPD Foundation, and infuses them with compassion and dedication to those whose lives are impacted by COPD. Now she has updated *Live Your Life with COPD - 52 Weeks of Health, Happiness, and Hope* with new chapters, stories, illustrations, expert Q & A, and more added insights. All of this, along with Jo-Von Tucker's timeless editorials and wise advice about life with COPD, make for an invaluable guide to daily living with COPD. This book is a roadmap to not just surviving, but thriving, with COPD and becoming your own COPD advocate.

If you have COPD or are a loved one or healthcare professional caring for those who do, you will benefit from reading this book. I know Jo-Von would be proud and smiling.

Celeste Belyea, RRT RN AE-C
Editor, The Pulmonary Paper

A Word from the Author

As I finish up my work on this book, we find ourselves in the midst of the Coronavirus (COVID-19) pandemic. At this time the best hope for controlling the spread of this potentially deadly disease rests in our ability to stay home and keep at least a six-foot distance between us and anyone who lives outside our own homes. In this book you'll find encouragement to get out of the house, meet new people, and do things you enjoy. Although it's simply not healthy, nor wise, at this time, to be physically close to others, we can still be in touch by phone, mail, and through the internet. Dear friends, keep your hearts and minds open to additional, creative ways to connect with others within the limitations we face. Stay well, keep the faith, and trust that "this too shall pass." Together, we will make our way through.

January – Week 1

Happy New Year!

"The successful man is one who had the chance and took it."

~ Roger Babson

A new year has begun, and with it, another opportunity to take control of our breathing – and our lives – with COPD. We enter a whole new year armed with actions we can take to improve our lung health; to stay active and fit, to follow our physician's treatment plan as prescribed, to strengthen our commitment to socialize and avoid isolation, and to look at that glass not as half empty, but always half full.

We have much to gain in this, making a New Year's resolution to breathe better. We can achieve a level of stability and remain well from day to day, as opposed to helplessly watching our health spin out of control and spiral into steady and swift decline! Stability for COPD'ers may appear fragile, but it doesn't have to be that way.

We can, and should, devote our energy to maintaining an active role in the management of our health. Side-by-side with our doctors and loved ones, we can be responsible for our health management – whatever is required to help balance our lives in our quest for improved health.

Our doctors can guide us, direct us, and measure our degree of success. Our family members can encourage and inspire us to be faithful with our regular exercise routine, take our medicines and to get the nutrition we need. They can even go along with us to doctors' appointments and support group meetings. Our respiratory therapists can help keep us on our toes regarding the proper use of supplemental oxygen and equipment, if it has been prescribed. They can test our oximetry to ensure we are receiving the maximum benefit from our O_2 (oxygen). And they will also most often be aware if we are using our oxygen as it has been prescribed for us.

Many people can be of help as we fight the good fight against COPD, but they can't do it for us! They can advise, they can cajole (although they shouldn't have to), and they can cheer from the sidelines whenever we've won a major battle with an exacerbation. But they cannot exercise for us, they cannot take our medicines for us, and they certainly cannot breathe for us! We are the ones who must be responsible for our accomplishments in health management!

So, you and me, let's make our New Year's Resolution right now – to commit ourselves to whatever it takes to have stability in our lives with COPD, to take control of our breathing – and our lives. We can do it. Now is the time.

Your Turn

Key points, or…if you don't remember anything else, remember this:

- Now is the time to make a fresh start.
- It is possible to take charge of your own health.
- You can be in control of your breathing – and your life.

Ask yourself this:

Have I ever made New Year's resolutions that were just too

overwhelming – and then when I couldn't follow through, it was discouraging?

This week:

Keep it simple. Make a promise to yourself to do at least three of the following things to improve your breathing – and stick with it! You can do as many as you want, but it's okay to pick only three. Just start somewhere.

- Tell yourself every day that you can learn to take control of your breathing.
- Commit to learning just one new thing each week from this book and put it into practice.
- Learn how your medicines work to open up your lungs. Different breathing medications work in different ways.
- Smile ten times every day.
- Start walking (approved by your doctor, of course), just one or two minutes at a time if that's all you can do. Add one more minute each day.
- Before you go to bed each night, write down something for which you are thankful.
- If you smoke, quit. If you fall down on it, don't be too hard on yourself. Get back up and try again.
- Wear your oxygen as prescribed. Every day.
- Try a new hobby or activity (or get back to something you were doing but stopped because of your breathing).

Great! You're on your way to taking charge of your health and breathing better. I'll check in with you in a few weeks to see how it's going.

January – Week 2

Know Your Numbers – Pulmonary Function Testing

"Education is learning what you didn't even know you didn't know."

~ Daniel Boorstin

Have you had your breathing tested and if so, do you know your numbers? You should!

Pulmonary function testing is a necessary part of diagnosing COPD. Your doctor wouldn't diagnose a patient with hypertension (high blood pressure) without taking a blood pressure reading or diagnose a patient with diabetes without ever assessing the blood sugar level. Just the same, if you have trouble breathing, or if you are at risk for COPD (see the questions at the end of this chapter) it's recommended to have a pulmonary function test. Once the results are in, you should know your numbers just as people with diabetes, high cholesterol, and high blood pressure know theirs.

There are two levels of pulmonary function testing: complete pulmonary function, and pulmonary function screen, or spirometry. A complete pulmonary function test takes about an hour. It measures flow (how the air moves through your bronchial airways), volume (how much air your lungs hold), resistance (how elastic or how stiff your lungs are), and diffusion (how well the oxygen moves from your lungs into your bloodstream). A pulmonary function screen, or spirometry, determines only the flow and volume of air moving in and out of your lungs. Spirometry takes a half hour or less.

The results of a spirometry test can provide information to you and your doctor about your ability to get your air out. It will help determine whether the problem with your lungs is obstructive (trouble getting the air out, as in COPD) or restrictive (trouble getting the air in). After your doctor has the results of your spirometry, he or she may order more tests – maybe a complete pulmonary function to understand more specifically what the problem is.

Your testing begins with determining your *normal predicted* lung function. The technician will ask questions such as, "What is your age, your gender, your height, your ethnicity?" The pulmonary function machine knows what the numbers would be for a person of your characteristics with perfectly healthy lungs. After the test your actual results are compared to the normal predicted. One test result for each maneuver is called *percent of normal predicted.* Here's an example: A person with perfectly healthy lungs who is your age, your height, your gender, and your ethnicity would normally exhale (blow out) two liters of air on a certain maneuver. If you are able to exhale only one liter, the result of that portion of the test would be 50% (half) of normal predicted. Test results of both spirometry and a complete pulmonary function will give your doctor and you many different numbers, each one pointing to your percent of normal predicted.

One key indicator of COPD is a decrease in FEV_1. This is the forced expiratory volume (how much air) you are able to breathe out in the first second of a long exhalation. Remember, when you have COPD, you have trouble getting your air *out*.

If you have COPD you should know your FEV_1 number and get a spirometry test regularly to watch for a decline in lung function. Although your lung function numbers, whether you have COPD or not, goes down with age, the goal is to maintain your numbers as much as possible and slow your progression of COPD. Although your

FEV_1 might vary a bit from year to year, if you have COPD, you cannot expect it to go up, even if you have an overall improvement in your ability to function in daily activities.

Talk with your doctor about having a spirometry test if you can answer "yes" to any of these questions. Do you have:

- Increased shortness of breath?
- Frequent coughing with or without mucus?
- Wheezing?
- Tightness in the chest?
- A history of smoking (cigarettes, pipes, cigars, etc.), second-hand smoke, fumes, chemicals, or dust in your work environment, or smoke from home cooking or heating fuel?
- A family history of COPD?

Added Insight

How to ask for spirometry – a question for Helen Sorenson

Q: I go to the doctor for breathing problems, but he does not say anything about ordering spirometry. What is the best way to go about asking for it without insulting my doctor?

A: If the doctor has already stated that you have COPD and you have never had spirometry done, ask, "Should I have further breathing tests performed?" If the doctor seems hesitant, say something like, "I'd like to know if my medicine is working and I understand breathing tests will give me numbers to go by."

If you had breathing tests done a long time ago, they should be repeated. Asking your doctor about spirometry may be a reminder that this needs to be done – he or she may just not realize it has been awhile since you were tested or may not be aware that you were NEVER tested.

If you have never had spirometry and you think you might have COPD or another breathing problem, show your doctor this chapter or have him/her visit the COPD Foundation website. If you bring your doctor credible information and are sincere, he or she should not be insulted.

Your Turn

Key points, or…if you don't remember anything else from this chapter, remember this:

- If you have trouble breathing, you should have your lung function tested.
- If you are diagnosed with COPD, you should know your FEV_1 number and what that means for you.

Ask yourself this:

- When is the last time I had spirometry?
- What is my FEV_1?

This week:

- Ask your doctor if you should have spirometry to check on the stability, or progression, of your COPD.
- If you've had a lung function test and don't know your FEV_1, ask your doctor.

January – Week 3

Your Relationship with Your Doctor

"It takes as much energy to wish as it does to plan."

~ Eleanor Roosevelt

If you have COPD, aside from the close relationships with your spouse and family members, the next most important person in your life is your doctor. How is your relationship with your primary care physician and/or your pulmonary specialist? Do you come away from checkups with your questions answered, satisfied with your medical treatment program, and feeling empowered in dealing with your situation? If not, perhaps you should take a good look at the relationship between you and your doctor. As you do, take a hard look at your own involvement too, much of what you do is at his or her advice.

As patients, we have a vital role to play in the management of our disease. We cannot fulfill that role if we are intimidated by the authority of doctors. Living day after day with a chronic disease, naturally, can cause us to feel vulnerable, especially if we have little knowledge of medicine. As patients, we must work at asserting ourselves and being self-confident, especially in interactions with our physicians. We should have equal roles of responsibility – letting the doctor know that we expect respect and consideration just as we give him or her the same in return.

We should tell our doctors, up front, that we'll do our best to follow the prescribed treatment plan. Yet, we must convey that we may have many questions in order to fully understand what is going on inside our lungs, what is required of us, and what the desired results should be. A good physician should welcome this approach; and a good doctor knows that the more we know about our disease, the better we can manage it and hold onto the highest quality of life possible. If your doctor says that you "ask too many questions," you may need to think about finding a new doctor – one who isn't threatened by questions, but accepts you as a patient who is eager to know what's going on. Our doctors should accept us as equal partners in the treatment of our own illness.

Doctors are busy and they keep a tight schedule. Here are some tips on how we can respect their time and get as much as we can from each appointment with them.

Seven Ways to Get the Most Out of Your Next Doctor Appointment

1. Think of your doctor as an equal partner in caring for your health – not someone who has all the answers, while you don't know anything.
2. Jot down questions in between appointments whenever you think of them. Keep them where you can find them and bring them to your next appointment.
3. Keep a separate folder or notebook to hold your health information: test results, a list of your current medications, and materials (in brief) that relate to your disease.
4. When you see your doctor, state your concerns clearly, taking just one to two minutes. You can say a lot in that time if you're organized! Tell him or her about changes in your breathing and your overall health since your last appointment.
5. Know what medications you're taking, their names, and what

they're supposed to do for your lungs. If you don't know, or if for instance, you aren't sure you're using your inhaled medications correctly – ask!

6. Be honest. Tell your doctor if you're still smoking and/or taking more puffs from your inhalers than prescribed.

7. Respect your doctor's time. Healthcare providers see a different patient every 15-30 minutes all day long and most of them are doing the very best they can to help you. Do your part to help them too.

Your Turn

Key points, or…if you don't remember anything else from this chapter, remember this…

- You and your doctor should be partners in managing your COPD.
- The more informed you are, the better you will be able to help yourself.
- Keep your health information together in a folder or notebook along with questions for your next appointment.

Ask yourself this:

- Does my doctor listen to what I'm trying to say?
- Am I organized in what I'm trying to say? Writing down two or three main points, helps.
- Do I feel comfortable asking my doctor questions? Don't worry about sounding silly. The only stupid question is the one you don't ask.

This week:

Make a list of questions about your lung function numbers and your level of disease. Keep in mind, though, if you ask the hard questions, you must be ready to take the answers.

Following up:

So, how are you doing on your New Year's resolutions? If you're still on track, good for you! Keep going! If you've fallen down a bit, don't beat yourself up about it. The important thing is to do *something* to help yourself breathe better. Don't give up! You can do it!

January – Week 4

Defying the Laws of Gravity... or... Holding on to Stability

"Take care of your body. It's the only place you have to live."

~ Jim Rohn

My number one commitment – my most important job – is to maintain stability of my disease. Except for a few exacerbations over the past fourteen years or so I've maintained a relatively stable condition. I've managed to avoid that slippery slope, the steady downward spiral that can happen to people with COPD. My FEV_1 (forced expiratory volume in the first second of exhalation, a major indicator of severity of COPD) has, until recently, remained mostly the same with small amounts of decline noted on lung function tests.

Staying stable takes a lot of commitment to my treatment program, and to staying as conditioned and active as I possibly can. The most difficult part of the search for stability, for me, has been getting enough rest. Working full time, coordinating a breathing support group, writing, editing, and publishing our monthly newsletter, and keeping up with volunteer work leaves me little time for resting and allowing my body to heal.

That's why the slippery slope of stability seems to me like defying the laws of gravity! Like a skilled trapeze artist from Cirque du Soleil, I've been able to ward off most lung infections, keeping my state of stability in the air at least temporarily, from one stretch to the next.

But like all good things, I suppose that combination of maneuverability and luck had to come to an end sometime. Kerplop! was the sound I seemed to hear as Dr. Mohr reported the latest results of my spirometry test. Gravity – 1, Jo-Von – 0. My lung function numbers had slipped precariously from 60% to about 45% within a short period of time.

Why? Several factors, probably – my age, exhaustion, and a general de-conditioning that has occurred since I was sick and hospitalized for a couple of weeks with colitis last fall. Altogether, a deadly combination that has definitely pulled me down to earth!

I share my personal experience only because I don't want to see it happen to you! We all work to hang on to our stability. I want my example to help you realize your own vulnerability, so you can take steps to preserve the quality of life you've established.

Why is this stability so important? Because once lost, it is extremely difficult to rebuild. Stamina and energy can be improved with the proper steps of management and treatment, but we must remember that our lungs do not regenerate. New replacement tissue will not grow. New functioning alveoli (tiny air sacs in the lungs where oxygen exchange takes place) will not appear – at least not yet, as scientists continue to work on it. You will naturally lose some lung function with time, even if you are successful at holding the disease at bay. Therefore, stability is precious! It is worth expending the effort to hold on to the highest level of COPD possible.

Here is what works for me. I'm passing these suggestions along with hopes that you can hold onto maximum stability as you fight your own battle with this thing we call COPD.

- Listen to your doctor! Understand the treatment program prescribed for you and follow it. Take your medications exactly as directed, including the use of supplemental oxygen.

- Be consistent with exercise. If you haven't participated in a pulmonary rehabilitation course, talk with your doctor about a referral. If you are a graduate of pulmonary rehab, consider taking a refresher course, or at least, continue your exercises and physical activities every day on your own.
- Be part of a breathing support group. Come, listen, talk, question, help, learn, share!
- Maintain social contact with the outside world. Do not let this disease rob you of interaction with friends, family, loved ones, and neighbors. Isolation leads to depression, and depression can lead to further debilitation.
- Pay attention to nutrition. Feed your body the right foods and nutrients to fuel it in the best way possible. Your body needs protein and a well-balanced diet of fruits, vegetables, meats, and dairy products. Ask your doctor about multi-vitamins. Take high-calorie supplements to put on weight, if necessary.
- Avoid exposure to viruses and cold germs. Wash your hands! Get the flu vaccine in the fall. Ask your doctor about getting a pneumonia vaccine booster if needed.
- Pay attention to changes such as a change in the color and/or consistency of your sputum, your regular cough routine, and your usual shortness of breath. (See information on the *My COPD Action Plan* at the end of this chapter.)
- Find the time to give your body the rest it needs. Do not push yourself to exhaustion. If you need an afternoon nap, take one. Listen to your body and do what it tells you to do when it needs a break.

Even if you take all these pro-active steps, you may still find it hard to achieve stability and maintain it. But it is well worth the effort. Remind yourself that no one can manage your disease for you!

It's something you have to do for yourself. That's why it's a good idea to keep a journal (see July – Week 4: Keeping a Journal) to write down your notes and thoughts about the ups and downs of your life with this disease. Keep track of good days and bad days, medicines you took, what seemed to help and what didn't. It can serve as a reminder when the situation comes up again.

The search for stability goes on. It may seem to you, too, as though you are trying to defy the laws of gravity. But remember, I've managed to accomplish stability for fourteen years. It took a series of negative circumstances to boot me off that tightrope, but I'm going to get back up there and give it all I've got to make my way to the other side – to stability.

Your Turn

Key points, or…if you don't remember anything else from this chapter, remember this:

- It's essential for a person with COPD to maintain stability.
- Follow the treatment plan your doctor and you have worked out.
- Know what is normal for you, pay attention when something has changed, and take action to stay well.

Ask yourself this:

- When was my last exacerbation?
- When was the one before that?

This week:

What new method or technique can I try this week that would add to what I already do to maintain stability with my COPD?

Here's more help:

- See chapter September – Week 3: Facing Fall – Preventing Exacerbations and When to Call the Doctor
- The *My COPD Action Plan* and *Report Exacerbations* card are available through a free download. www.copdfounda-tion.org

January – Week 5

Reclaiming Your Life through Pulmonary Rehabilitation

"The important thing is somehow to begin."

~ Henry Moore

One of the biggest issues you, as a person with COPD may be facing, is the loss of your former level of activity: loss of the ability to do what you used to do, and perhaps the biggest of all, the loss of control over your breathing, and your life. Pulmonary rehabilitation can help you regain strength and control and give you a new start to living well with COPD.

What is pulmonary rehab? Here are those six classic questions: Who, what, when, where, why, and how, and their answers.

Who should go?

Should I participate in pulmonary rehab? Discuss this with your doctor if you can answer "yes" to any of the following questions.

- Do you have COPD and are becoming less physically active?
- Have you had to give up or cut back on activities because of changes brought on by changes in your breathing?
- Are you feeling tired and short of breath (SOB) more often?
- Do you find yourself having frequent bouts of bronchitis,

pneumonia, or being down with a bad cold for longer periods of time than other people your age?

- Are you confused about your breathing medications, unsure if they're working or not?
- Do you feel downhearted because of your decline in breathing and activity?

What is it?

Pulmonary rehabilitation is a program of exercise and education especially designed for people with COPD and other chronic lung diseases. In pulmonary rehab you'll gain strength, stamina, and flexibility, while learning a lot about your lungs and how to stay as healthy as possible. You'll also find moral support and learn to cope with changes brought on by COPD.

In addition to this, it is important to note what pulmonary rehab *cannot* do. Pulmonary rehab cannot cure your lung disease (there is currently no cure for COPD), cannot improve your lung function numbers, or make you feel like you're twenty again!

However, pulmonary rehab *can* improve your overall physical conditioning (conditioned muscles require less oxygen) and show you how you can be less likely to have COPD exacerbations. Pulmonary rehab can help you learn to breathe effectively and control your breathing during shortness of breath episodes. In addition to physical conditioning, effective lung health management, and breathing control, you'll find ways to cope with lung disease and live your life as fully as possible.

Participants in pulmonary rehab often learn the best lessons from each other. After all, they're traveling the same road. Participants often say, "This is the only place I can come where everybody understands what I'm going through."

You might be thinking, "Okay, this sounds all well and good, but I have never been one to exercise. To be honest, I'm kind of scared. What will they make me do in pulmonary rehab?" While specifics vary, here are the basic components of pulmonary rehab.

Health history

You'll sit down with a nurse and/or a respiratory therapist and tell them about your health history. Yes, they will ask if you smoked and if you are still smoking. But, the professionals at pulmonary rehab know that it's really hard to quit. They're there to help you, not to place blame.

Six-minute walk

You'll walk with a therapist or nurse while having your oxygen level, heart rate, and blood pressure monitored. The point of the six-minute walk is to see how much distance you can cover in six minutes. Don't worry if you can't walk far. That's why you're there!

Warm up stretches and strengthening

You may work with sticks, resistance bands, and/or light hand weights.

Exercise equipment

Bikes, arm ergometers (arm peddlers), treadmills, and recumbent steppers are some of the equipment you'll have the option to use. Remember, the staff at pulmonary rehab specializes in working with people who are short of breath. They'll help you find the best way to exercise in a way that is safe and comfortable.

Class sessions

You'll learn about breathing techniques, medications, nutrition, pacing, conserving energy, relaxation, stress management, developing coping skills, and more.

When would I go?

Pulmonary rehab usually takes place two to three times per week with each session lasting an hour or two. Your time in the program will last from six to twelve weeks, depending on the program. Some programs offer a continuing maintenance phase in which you may continue after graduation and come for as long as you want. Many people continue for years in this affordable self-pay phase.

Where will I find a pulmonary rehab program?

Pulmonary rehab programs are commonly found in hospital buildings and clinics. (Don't worry, pulmonary rehabilitation is an out-patient program and usually not located near in-patient areas of the hospital.) Some programs are located in fitness centers and store fronts.

Why should I go to pulmonary rehab?

Here are some of the results you can expect if you participate. You will:

- Learn about COPD and how to manage it.
- Learn how to breathe more effectively, moving more air with less effort.
- Learn how you can be less likely to require emergency room visits and hospital admissions due to breathing problems.
- Be in better overall physical condition with more stamina and flexibility.
- Learn coping skills for dealing with your COPD.
- Learn how to avoid anxiety, panic, and feelings of depression related to your breathing.
- Have fun while finding friendship and support, knowing you're not alone!

How do I start?

Medicare requires that you have a written referral from your physician. Check with your health insurer for requirements specific to your policy.

Added Insight

Nick's story

A self-described "farm boy" Nick Wilkinson grew up in rural West Michigan during The Great Depression. After serving in the Air Force in World War II he returned home, married, and became the father of four children. Nick worked in the farm implement business, eventually owning a share in his family's company. From time to time Nick noticed that some things in his environment such as dust, mold, and humidity caused his breathing to feel "tight." All the while he smoked cigarettes. Like so many people Nick smoked for a long time and never thought it would catch up with him. Here is his story about how pulmonary rehab gave him help and hope.

It was a warm summer night. Nick was having a lot of trouble breathing and didn't know what to do. He had a horrible, suffocating feeling, and was wondering if each breath would be his last. Nick was rushed by ambulance to the hospital emergency room. There he had X-rays, breathing treatments, and other medications, as well as arterial blood gases (ABG's), a test that shows the oxygen level in the blood.

The infection that affected Nick's breathing that terrible night eventually went away, but the challenges he faced from COPD had just begun. Although he was able to quit smoking, he described his breathing over the next few years as "a struggle" at best. He seemed to be doing less but becoming more tired and short of breath. These changes prompted Nick's wife, Blanche, to have concern for her husband, a man who had been so strong and healthy, who she now saw struggling so hard just to breathe.

When Nick walked into the pulmonary rehab department he told the staff softly, "My doctor thinks this program will help, and my wife wants me to come, but I don't know if there's anything you people can do to help me." As Nick began participating in the program, he remained skeptical. Back then he thought his inhalers were doing him more harm than good, he didn't believe that a pulse oximeter really worked, and couldn't imagine how pursed-lips breathing could help.

Nevertheless, with Blanche at his side, Nick drove twenty-five miles one way twice a week (in the West Michigan winter!) to participate in exercise and education. Gradually Nick's exercise capacity increased along with his confidence in what was being taught to him by the staff. He felt so much better and had more control over his breathing, rather than feeling as if his breathing had control over him.

"Before this program, I didn't know *what* to do to help myself. But here I learned how to use my inhalers and found out that they really do work. I've also learned to live with my lung condition."

"A big part of it is that he's learned to cope," added Blanche.

Before coming to the program Nick didn't know how to avoid breathing troublemakers or how to watch for the early warning signs of a bad episode. "I've learned how to think ahead and not get myself into these circumstances. It's also helped a lot to work with my doctor and be able to ask questions. And I've learned that exercise helps. Pulmonary rehab has definitely been worth the time and effort. It really has."

Nick went on to continue in the maintenance phase of pulmonary rehab, faithfully attending exercise every week while having fun and making new friends in class. A goal of his was to start bowling again, which he did! Nick also rediscovered the joy of driving his tractor and traveling with Blanche. Knowing how much participating in pulmonary rehab had helped him breathe better, feel better, and live better, Nick became one of the program's biggest promoters. He encouraged friends and acquaintances with COPD to live better by joining pulmonary rehab.

Often after exercise class Nick would pause a few minutes to talk privately with staff. He would put his hand on a staff member's shoulder, sincerely and emotionally saying, "You people have helped me so much. I just want to see others have the chance to improve like I have."

INSPIRATION

This acrostic poem was created by a classmate in Nick's pulmonary rehab class.

I love Pulmonary Rehab

N umber One: Get involved!

S pecial instructors

P eople who encourage each other

I t makes me feel healthy

R eally having fun

A ttitude makes the difference

T otal dedication

I t has made me a believer. Exercise works!

O ngoing participation keeps me strong

N ever give up!

Your Turn

Key points, or…if you don't remember anything else from this chapter, remember this:

- Pulmonary rehabilitation cannot fix your lungs.
- It can help you improve your endurance, strength, and flexibility.
- It can show you how to stay as healthy as possible, even with COPD, as well as provide encouragement and support.

Ask yourself this:

Am I ready to give this a try?

This week:

Ask your doctor if he or she would consider referring you to pulmonary rehabilitation.

February – Week 1

Your Relationship with Others and the Need to Love, and Be Loved

*The better you know yourself, the better your re-
lationship with the rest of the world.*

~ Toni Collette

*"When skies are sunny or when skies are gray-
Remember your inhaler when LOVE takes your breath away.*

~ Stephanie Williams

Those of us with COPD may not be aware of the impact our disease has on those around us, especially those closest to us – spouse,
friends, and family. We often find ourselves more dependent on others as the disease progresses, and we find we're unable to continue
equal sharing in household responsibilities. The small chores we've
always done are no longer within our scope of abilities, due to shortness of breath.

When this happens, we may become angry, hurt, and resentful.
Our spouses and/or family members might also harbor anger and
resentment without even knowing it. One person becomes angry
at being so dependent, and the other is angry about becoming so

depended upon. Added to this is guilt; guilt on the part of the person with COPD because of feelings of inadequacy for having to rely so heavily on the other party; and guilt on the part of the partner for resenting the added responsibilities.

To help, or not to help?

No matter how physically limited the person with COPD may be, excessive dependency or doting, should be discouraged. It's alright for people with lung disease to push their restrictions and boundaries as much as safely possible, and frequently they will need encouragement to do so. In this case, "use it or lose it" does apply.

On the other hand, the wife, husband, or partner of the person with COPD needs to be sensitive to signs of frustration and over-exertion. These are signs that may be silently coming from their mate who could be in denial, and showing it, by tackling chores that are clearly beyond their physical abilities. Sometimes the person with COPD may try to express themselves through non-verbal communication with distressed looks, signaling their partner to just read their mind. The "can't-you-see-I'm-struggling-here?" message is sent. But it truly is unfair to expect someone else to read our thoughts.

This kind of misunderstanding happens with close friends and family members, as well. Communication is the key to understanding and acceptance of our restrictions. This is true and applies to all of our relationships: as couples, friends, parents, siblings, or even distant cousins! It is much better to clearly communicate our needs and wishes than it is to risk misunderstood actions and statements.

Communication

It helps to tell our friends up front about our limitations, rather than trying to hide them. We can do so without dwelling on the issue, simply by stating our situation. Conduct open discussions with your spouse about household chores, schedules, and shared responsibilities; adjustments can be made as needed. Modifications can even make some activities more physically possible than before, such as saying, "Maybe if we just do it this way...let's try it and see how it works."

It's essential to be open and straightforward about our restrictions. But if we still find that our partner is less understanding than we would like, we should check our own behavior and communication skills. There may be room for improvement there, too. It helps to ask peers in our breathing support group, pulmonary rehab class, or online support group how they would handle a particular situation. Then we can talk openly and frankly with our partners about expectations on *both* sides.

As individuals with COPD, we must work hard to maintain self-esteem as we battle our way through the ravages of this disease. When we're successful in communicating as we maintain quality of life – albeit somewhat altered – and when we manage our disease as effectively as possible, we will project an attitude of self-respect. And that is clearly received by those around us – with the same kind of respect sent right back to us. We can then deal effectively with the many emotional issues facing us and be a better mate in spite of our disease.

The need to love and be loved

Even if you communicate, though, you may still find that having COPD can make it hard to feel lovable. We don't feel well, we don't think we look very good, we can't do what we once could, and we often sense that we're on the outside of a normal, healthy world looking in.

In spite of our COPD, though, we must hold on to believe that we are loved, and lovable. This might be one of the most challenging aspects of living with COPD. But we must be self-affirming, and able to trust in those around us and believe in the love, care, and respect that we receive. With or without COPD we often tend to be less caring of ourselves than of those around us. Frankly, if we loved our friends and family the way we love ourselves, they'd receive pretty shoddy treatment. At the same time, the less we value ourselves, the harder it is to share loving feelings with others.

It's a basic human need to love and be loved, and if that need is not met, we become stressed. This type of stress can cause us to withdraw from those around us and turn in on ourselves, as we are less active and short of breath. Loneliness can lead to further focus on our ailments, until our lives are ruled by an almost obsessive preoccupation with our body, its functions and malfunctions. Of course, we should be mindful of signs and symptoms of COPD problems, but it is dangerous to be overly preoccupied with our condition.

Unfortunately, there are those whose own problems keep them from loving us, and in this case, we may consider spending less time with them – or avoiding them altogether. We can't fix everybody and everything. We can't solve everybody's problems. We have to love ourselves and we have to take care of ourselves, and this includes steering clear of negativity.

Giving of ourselves – our feelings, hopes, and dreams despite fears of misunderstanding and rejection, builds the kind of intimacy that relieves the stress of isolation and the agony of disease. Loving others, caring for their needs, surprising them – even delighting them – gives our own lives meaning. To give of ourselves in this way requires that we value ourselves and trust that a word or action from us could bring joy to someone. Even with COPD, we have the power within us to raise someone's spirits, to make his or her day brighter. The healing power of helping others is amazing and serves us well. We must have the courage to give freely of ourselves and know in our hearts that the love and trust we accord to others will be returned in kind.

Romance and intimacy – really?

Finally, a word to those of you who have a significant other – a romantic partner – in your life. You may be concerned that COPD will keep you from expressing yourself intimately with that special person. Know that just because you're short of breath, that doesn't mean that you can't engage in sexual intimacy and benefit from the closeness and enjoyment it brings. It may take some changes and adjustments, but you can be intimate. Hugging, touching, and caressing can be satisfying in expressing love with your partner. Talk about it. Feel free to talk, also, with your doctor, nurse, respiratory therapist, or counselor about ways to do this. If they can't help you, hopefully they will refer you to someone who can.

Having COPD can bring on many changes in your life and the lives of those near and dear to us. But, my friends, do your best to love and respect yourself. Then accept my wish that the love and care you show to others will come back around to you.

Your Turn

Key points, or…if you don't remember anything else from this chapter, remember this:

- When you have COPD, communication is essential to enjoying a good relationship with others.
- If you have COPD, try to do what you can to contribute to life at home. But don't be afraid to ask for help.
- If you are a caregiver/well spouse for a person with COPD, allow that person to do all they can to help around the house. Don't dote on them.
- As human beings, we have the need to love and be loved in spite of COPD.

- Respect and love yourself.
- Sexual expression comes in many forms and is possible to achieve with COPD, even if you have significant shortness of breath.

Ask yourself this:

- Do I, or my partner, have feelings of resentment and guilt regarding the changes brought on by COPD?
- Do I have a loving relationship with somebody – a spouse, family member, or close friend – who appreciates me? Do I regularly spend time with him or her?

This week:

- If there is tension in your relationships, talk about it. Begin with "I feel…" instead of "you do…" or "you don't…" Using this method is non-accusatory – and nobody can ever take it away when you state, "I feel…"
- Call that special person, send a card or flowers, and tell them they mean a lot to you.

Here's more help:

National Jewish Health has excellent, detailed information on relationships and intimacy with COPD. https://www.nationaljewish. org/conditions/copd-chronic-obstructive-pulmonary-disease/over-view/lifestyle-management/living-with-chronic-lung-disease/intima-cy 1.877.225.5654

February – Week 2

COPD Research

"Cutting off fundamental, curiosity-driven science is like eating the seed corn. We may have a little more to eat next winter but what will we plant so we and our children will have enough to get through the winters to come?"

~ Carl Sagan

Thank you to the research team at the COPD Foundation for their help with this chapter.

Whenever we hear about a specific disease, it's only natural to assume that there is ongoing research to find a cure, or at least a way to manage symptoms. We wonder if there are any positive results from all the data collected and, if so, how long it might be before help is available to all patients. Unfortunately, COPD-related research has not made as much progress as other diseases.

COPD is currently the fourth leading cause of death in the U.S. and worldwide. Knowing this, you might think that funding for research would be similar to that of other prevalent diseases. Sadly, this is not the case. According to ClinicalTrials.gov, there are 690 ongoing trials for COPD in contrast to over 36,000 trials taking place in cancer research!* This is certainly not to say that cancer and other chronic diseases should have less research, but, that COPD research should be more common – and better funded.

Yet, this remains an exciting time for COPD. Despite the limited funding, progress is being made to enhance COPD research.

Source: ClinicalTrials.gov, May 3, 2020.

COPD PPRN

It is estimated that more than 300 million individuals worldwide have COPD. Unfortunately, historically there has been no central resource to connect people interested in participating in COPD research with COPD researchers. To address this need, the COPD Patient-Powered Research Network (COPD PPRN) was established. The COPD PPRN (www.copdpprn.org) is a registry of individuals who have been diagnosed with chronic obstructive pulmonary disease or may be at risk for developing COPD. The COPD PPRN is the largest network of patients affected by chronic obstructive pulmonary disease (COPD) ever assembled, and provides an opportunity for people diagnosed with COPD and those at risk for COPD, to join a community of individuals who want to revolutionize COPD research.

Individuals enrolled in the COPD PPRN have agreed to share their health information and may, at some point, be asked if they would be willing to participate in clinical research studies. Information in the COPD PPRN is kept in a secure database to be used exclusively for research. COPD PPRN participants do not have to take part in research studies, *as participation in all clinical trials is voluntary*. Each individual is free to decide what's best for them.

Overseen by a patient-led governing board, the COPD PPRN is unique, and patient centered. If you're looking for a way to make a difference, consider enrolling in the COPD PPRN.

COPD Biomarkers Qualification Consortium

The COPD Biomarkers Qualification Consortium was formed in 2010 to help fast track research for better treatment and medicines that will help improve the lives of those with COPD.

What are biomarkers and Clinical Outcome Assessments (COAs)?

A biomarker is something that can be tested and measured and provides an indication of normal biological processes. Among other things, it could be an element in a blood test, x-ray or other bodily measurement. A clinical outcome describes or reflects how an individual feels, functions or survives, such as a mark of achievement in a physical activity or a score on a survey. The results of these tests and measures can help determine if a person has a certain disease, and if particular treatments work to reduce symptoms or exacerbations, or to slow progression.

What is a consortium, and why is it needed?

A consortium is a group of companies or organizations that pool their resources to achieve a common goal. It is needed because, although some COPD research data exists, it is spread out in many places within different groups and organizations: pharmaceutical companies, academic research centers, the National Heart Lung and Blood Institute and other groups of researchers. By having this data in one place, there may be enough information for biomarkers to meet the requirements of the Food and Drug Administration (FDA) and other regulatory agencies such as the European Medicines Agency (EMA). These organizations could then use the biomarkers and COAs to evaluate new treatments. So far, the COPD biomarkers consortium has been successful, with the first biomarker and the first COA for COPD approved by the FDA. The consortium continues work on several other biomarkers and clinical assessment tools.

COPDGene® Study

COPDGene is one of the largest studies ever funded by the National Heart, Lung and Blood Institute (NHLBI) of the National Institutes of Health. This study aims to find inherited or genetic factors that make some people more likely to develop COPD.

COPDGene also works to classify different types of COPD and understand how the disease may vary from person to person. The study's advancements include the identification of genes that relate to the risk of causing COPD, and which groups of people are at high risk for disease progression.

Involving other aspects of COPD

According to the FDA, most of the treatments in use for COPD focus on improving airway obstruction in order to help you exhale easier with less wheezing. While this is important, there are other significant health impacts of COPD. Consideration of these aspects of COPD can help shape some research moving forward and hopefully lead to the discovery of new therapies that will improve the overall health of people with COPD. These therapies could stop or slow exacerbation episodes, or they could even slow the progression of the disease.

Of course, we'd all like to see more changes – major changes – in the treatment and management of COPD. And it's easy to understand that for many of you, change can't come fast enough. But the important message is that progress is being made! The groundwork for expanding research has been laid. More individuals impacted by COPD are becoming involved every day, and most importantly, they have a voice in deciding how to direct research, so it focuses on the needs of patients. Consider getting involved and becoming part of the solution.

What about stem cell therapy?

You may be wondering about stem cell therapy and if there are any research studies going on with that. Please see chapter September – Week 2 for information.

Your Turn

Key points, or...If you don't remember anything else, remember this:

- COPD is the fourth leading cause of death in the U.S. and worldwide.
- There are 780 ongoing COPD-related research trials compared to over 41,000 trials taking place in cancer research. More research is needed.
- The COPD PPRN connects COPD researchers and people interested in participating in COPD research (www.copdpprn. org).

Ask yourself this:

Am I looking for a way to make a difference? Should I consider enrolling in the COPD PPRN?

This week:

Visit the COPD Foundation website: www.copdfoundation.org and click on "Research."

Here's more help:

For a list of COPD research currently taking place, go to: www.clinicalconnection.com/.

February – Week 3

Good Days, Bad Days

"This, too, shall pass."

~ William Shakespeare

One of the most puzzling aspects in life with COPD is the fact that we have good days, as well as bad days. One day we feel pretty darn good, able to greet the day and do what we want to do. The next day, we find ourselves struggling to breathe with the slightest exertion. Have you heard of a "bad hair day"? This is a "bad air" day – and it's most frustrating because it's bad for no obvious reason. It just is – and we all have them.

Worsened shortness of breath is usually the first sign of a bad day. In my own case this is always accompanied by debilitating fatigue, an overwhelming tiredness that makes every little activity a major chore. For our caregivers, spouses, and family members, this is a touchy subject that as COPD'ers, we can't explain. No wonder it's hard for those around us to understand!

What causes those bad days? Why do we feel relatively well one day and the next, suddenly take a turn for the worse? Is the barometric pressure changing? Is it pollen in the air? Is an infection brewing? (To learn the early warning signs of a lung infection, see chapter September – Week 3: Facing Fall – Preventing Exacerbations and When to Call the Doctor.) Did we overexert yesterday? Have we been around someone with a cold or flu virus? Has our diet changed? Are we emotionally upset about something? Is the humidity too high? The list goes on and on.

Our choices of ways to deal with those bad days are narrowed considerably by our physical limitations. But deal with them, we must. These are the times we need to call forth all the coping skills we possess. Although there are no magic, quick cures for making us feel better, there are ways to get through the bad times.

One of the most important things we can do for ourselves, whether we are fighting an infection or just dealing with a bad day, is to allow extra time for rest. We should always make sure we get enough sleep. A restless night can cause us to feel badly the next day, so a little catch-up time is probably in order. Peaceful sleep helps us build up our reserves after a bout of illness.

If you are one of those individuals who simply cannot sleep in the daytime, be sure to get additional rest, limit your physical exertion, and deliberately plan activities that you can do while seated or lying down. Maybe there's a book you've been meaning to read, a jigsaw puzzle to put together, or a sit-down fix-it project to do. A bad day may give you the opportunity to still get something done and save your energy as you do.

Watch your diet on the bad days. Avoid gassy foods such as carbonated soda, beans, and Brussels sprouts. The gas pushes up on your diaphragm, making it even harder to breathe. If you're not on a fluid restriction because of your heart, drink plenty of fluids – water is best – and go easy on the caffeine. If you tend to retain fluid in your feet and ankles, ask your doctor if you should sit with your feet propped up for fifteen minutes or so, a few times on that day. Eat regular, balanced meals, even if they are small ones.

Be sure to take your medications as prescribed. If your doctor's order is to use your fast-acting rescue medication up to four-times a day, but you don't usually need it, this is a good day for it. Open up your lungs as best you can. They're telling you they need it!

Save multiple projects for the good days that will surely follow the bad ones. It isn't wise to tax your already stressed system by trying to keep too many balls in the air at once. It's hard enough to juggle time and needs, even when you feel pretty good.

Lastly, deal with your bad days by seeking ways of bringing joy into your life. Find things that make you laugh. It's hard to feel bad when you have tears of laughter rolling down your face! If you find joy in listening to music, take time for it. Music can be a wonderful diversion from having to work for each breath. And let's remind ourselves that those elusive good days are not far away. If we can just get past the bad one that looms over us now, things will surely improve.

So, grab that favorite pillow, the teddy bear that nobody else knows about, a good book, or a funny movie, and tuck in for a healing time. Do it before you get those eyes-to-the-ceiling looks from those around you, and before you affect their day. Calmly state that you are having a bad day and hope they will accept that. It all works together to make your life more bearable right then and there!

Here's wishing you far more good days than bad ones!

Added Insight I

How the weather affects breathing

In respiratory therapist Sandy Wright's pulmonary rehab class, when her COPD patients were discouraged about their "bad air" days, she put them to work, not with a new routine on treadmills and bicycles, but in a different way. Sandy began by explaining that the weather can have a lot to do with bad breathing days, and to help them see this for themselves she suggested they conduct a study.

"I told them to watch the local weather reports every day and track the humidity, the barometric pressure, and the dew point, and also to document how they were breathing on that day.

"The results showed that some of my patients were more affected by the humidity while others were more affected by the dew point, which they were surprised about. The higher the dew point, the harder it was to breathe even if the other [weather] indicators were within normal limits.

"So that was it in a nutshell. After this, they better understood that weather had something to do with their breathing. With this information they could plan their day accordingly and not get upset if they were having a bad breathing day. They knew it would pass and it wasn't that their COPD was getting worse."

Added Insight II

Morning Body Scan, Mindful meditation -- Jo-Von Tucker

We just talked about ups and downs – good days and bad days – with COPD. To make those bad air days as good as possible we must listen to our bodies. Having a positive attitude helps to even out the peaks and valleys of energy and wellness but communicating with our inner self is the best way of tuning in to see what's in store.

One helpful coping skill involves mindful meditation. Here are some ways to work towards mindful meditation. Try surrounding yourself with quiet serenity. If you're having a rotten day, try to get away from noise and bustling activity. If you can, create some alone time in a quiet room with peaceful music; watch a movie on TV or your computer; or just drive to the beach or other tranquil, scenic place.

Mindful meditation also means emptying your mind of all extraneous thoughts and focusing on your body to help you control your shortness of breath. Deep breathing will get you to the right point of concentration. If you haven't mastered this magnificent tool of relaxation yet, give it a try.

Mindful meditation is the art of listening to the status of our bodies. We can tap into the state of our bodies even before we rise from bed in the morning. Here's something that works for me, and I recommend you give it a try. *As always, check with your doctor to make sure that any new physical activity is safe for you.*

When you awaken, take a few minutes to stretch like a lazy cat, reaching your hands high over your head and pointing the tips of your toes downward. Repeat this a couple of times with pursed-lips breathing.

Then start to relax and close your eyes again – don't fall back asleep! Breathe deeply and steadily, focusing on your breathing. When you feel nice and relaxed, focus on the tips of your toes. Visualize first your toes, then slowly your entire feet, as being free of pain and stiffness.

Work your way up with your mind focused next on your ankles, then your calves. In your mind, breathe any pain or stiffness right out of them. Spend a good bit of time thinking about your knees; your joints just may need extra concentration.

Slowly scan your body as you work your way up to the top of your head. Leave no major muscles and bones untouched by your scan. Just like an X-ray or an MRI, you can scan your body a little bit at a time to check for illness or pain. Then visualize each stopping place as the spot to rid yourself of pain, or at least acknowledge that it is there to be dealt with.

You may find you'll need a lot of practice to become proficient with mindful meditation. That's okay. The better you get at scanning your body in your mind, the quicker you can ascertain your good day/ bad day status.

My friends, remember this: If you find, after your morning body scan, that you are headed full tilt for a bad day, it doesn't mean that you must give in to its demands. You don't have to like it, but you can co-exist. Instead of being angry and fighting it, simply recognize that it exists. Finally, know that a positive attitude goes a long way toward easing your way through until you wake up tomorrow, hopefully to a better day.

Your Turn

Key points, or…if you don't remember anything else from this chapter, remember this:

- Frustrating as it may be, good days and bad days without reason, are a fact of life with COPD.
- When having a bad air day always check if you have early warning signs of a lung infection (chapter September – Week 3: Facing Fall – Preventing Exacerbations and When to Call the Doctor).
- Don't push yourself on the bad days, but take it easy, even if you have to postpone plans.
- If possible, do something enjoyable on a bad air day.

Ask yourself this:

- How did I spend my most recent bad air day?
- Should I do something different next time?

This week:

- Set aside fun or interesting sit-down projects – something you will enjoy doing – for your next bad air day.

Here's more help:

Make a brief call to a friend or log on to an online support group to express that you're having a bad day. Keep it brief. Your friends with COPD will understand and help you get through it. The COPD Foundation's online community is COPD360social. https://www.copd-foundation.org COPD360social/Community/Activity-Feed.aspx

February – Week 4
Panic and Anxiety in COPD

"The first rule is to keep an untroubled spirit. The second is to look things in the face and know them for what they are."

~ Marcus Aurelius

Anxiety and panic are common in COPD. It's been found that those with COPD have substantially higher odds of generalized anxiety disorder (GAD) compared to those without COPD. Let's start with looking at comments from some people with COPD who have had problems with anxiety and/or panic attacks. Perhaps you'll find something that sounds familiar. To protect their identity, assumed names are used.

Julia
I must be having some sort of breakdown as I am constantly sad, worried, and live in fear each and every day. I fear getting up each morning because I am fearful of feeling not well again. I cannot enjoy my family because I feel I am not part of their life anymore as I am always not well. I cannot enjoy food or social life. I have become almost reclusive as I fear becoming breathless and spoil my partner's time out. I find myself constantly holding my breath and fear that my COPD is raging on. The more breathless and anxious I feel, the more I notice myself holding my

breath. I feel there is no quality of life.

Sorry for moaning but I can't seem to get in control. Exercise is proving difficult as I am anxious of becoming more breathless, which in turn makes it harder for me to manage my life. I fear living, as I feel very isolated and trapped in this body that doesn't work. My aim is to try to be more positive and take each day as it comes, and focusing on myself and my well-being, hopefully without fear.

John

I think my panic attacks result from not getting enough oxygen in my system. Don't confuse this with a normal person panting for breath and hyperventilating. Not the same thing. Panic and anxiety are feelings I have when I can't get my breath. Then I begin to tense up, feeling over-whelmed, jittery, and very nervous.

Don

My heart races, I get sweaty, and I am short of breath when I move around. I am on O_2 [supplemental oxygen] when I am up doing things. I sometimes wonder – possibly atrial fibrillation [irregular heartbeat]? Should I get a sleep study done or ask my doctor if I should wear a heart monitor for 24 hours or more? My friend told me I may even need an "event monitor" to monitor any suspicious heart activity. Could it be a combination of all the meds I take? I do try to stay calm and use the PLB (pursed-lips breathing). Sometimes it works and sometimes it doesn't. What else I can do?

Rodney

My O_2 sats [oxygen saturations] go up and down. I am now on O_2 at bedtime and lately when I am out and about, I am getting these really *bad panic attacks. I wake up in the middle of the night with panicky feelings and have a hard time trying to fall asleep. Is there anything I can do to lessen these feelings?*

COPD has many faces. Yet, there are challenges, doubts, hopes, and fears we all share.

John may have a tendency to be more anxious than Don. Julia might have had an anxiety disorder before she was ever diagnosed with a breathing disorder. Don might have more concerns about his COPD symptoms or additional signs related to other medical conditions, than Rodney.

Two people with the same degree of breathlessness, or shortness of breath (SOB), may differ regarding the extent to which it bothers them. One person might say, "I am having trouble breathing," while another may experience an alarming sensation, thinking, "I will die of suffocation." Each will store these experiences in their memory differently, setting different levels of apprehension and anticipatory anxiety. One might remember it simply as a discomforting experience, which is a nuisance that can be managed. Another may remember it as "I could have died" or "I felt I was going to die. I never want to go through that again." Some, when anxious, hold their breath or start breathing rapidly, and some seem to feel the chest tightening and throat closing more than others do. These are all variations of normal human response to our perception of danger or threat of harm.

Experiencing anxiety, as well as depression, does not mean you are "weak" or "going crazy." Actually, the presence of anxiety or depression shows, simply, that you are human and react like a normal human being. Seeking help or accepting treatment does not mean, "I've lost control, I have failed" or "I am falling apart." Seeking help when one needs it is the wise thing to do.

Breathlessness can cause anxiety and anxiety can increase breathlessness. The more anxious we feel about breathing, the worse the breathlessness gets. COPD, with or without anxiety or depression, can also affect family relationships and participation in social life, even as far as self-imposed isolation from your partner and family, and losing all interest and joy in relating to others.

There is help and hope! Here are some things you can do if you have panic and anxiety with COPD:

1. Make sure you have been tested thoroughly for lung function and heart function.
2. When you and your doctor know the physical cause of your discomfort and have taken the necessary steps to regain and maintain your health, you may need an assessment for anxiety, and subsequently learn coping skills. Discuss this with your doctor and be honest about how you feel.
3. You may benefit from anxiety reduction breathing techniques such as pursed-lips breathing and abdominal, or diaphragmatic (DB), breathing. These techniques can be taught by a respiratory therapist (or a physical or occupational therapist specializing in respiratory issues) along with activity and exercise. Learn these techniques and use them to manage and control anxiety.
4. Physical and mental relaxation can be a powerful tool for dealing with breathlessness and anxiety. Learn relaxation skills. Relax tense muscles, anxious thoughts, and an anxious mind.
5. Your doctor may prescribe an anxiety medication. These medications do help, and you should not hesitate to try them.
6. Ask your doctor if you should talk to a counselor or other mental health specialist. It is not a sign of weakness to talk with somebody about issues that affect your health, happiness, and well-being.

Panic and anxiety are common in people with COPD. Breathlessness can cause anxiety and anxiety can increase shortness of breath. The more anxious we feel about breathing, the worse the breathlessness gets. But there is help, and there is a lot you can do to feel better if you have panic and anxiety with COPD.

Your Turn

Key points, or…if you don't remember anything else from this chapter, remember this:

- It is normal to have feelings of panic and anxiety with COPD.
- Reactions to feelings of panic and anxiety differ from person to person.
- Make sure you and your doctor have ruled out physical causes such as heart disease, which can also trigger feelings of panic and anxiety.
- Learning correct breathing techniques along with other treatments and methods, can help you control panic and anxiety in COPD.

Ask yourself this:

- Do I sometimes feel panic and/or anxiety because of my COPD?
- If so, what happened the last time I felt this way?

This week:

Plan and practice what you will do if you have an episode of panic and/or anxiety. If you don't know where to start, ask your doctor about getting help.

March – Week 1

Panic Attack! The Anatomy and Physiology of a Panic Attack

*"It's not so much what we know as how
well we use what we know."*

~ Ernesta Procope

This is not intended as medical advice. Show this information to your doctor. Together you can develop a plan that works best when you begin to feel panic and anxiety with COPD.

What causes a panic attack? In this chapter we're going to talk about what happens, physically, how symptoms are interconnected, and what causes symptoms to escalate into a full-blown panic attack. Once you understand how a panic attack starts and builds, you will hopefully be able to forestall the onset, or at least modify the intensity of symptoms. As you acquire further knowledge and skills in this area, you may be able to stop them altogether.

A panic attack is nothing but the body's emergency system at work! This system swings into action by an alarm (often a false alarm) set off by your brain. Breath dysregulation (problem with the regulation of breathing) may be the major reason for setting off the emergency alarm or, let's say, our "panic button."

Because breathing problems are a major part of panic attacks, sorting out what's really going on is particularly tricky for people with heart and lung disease. You hear a lot about the anatomy of the lungs: airways, air sacs, diaphragm, accessory muscles, etc., in connection with breathing. But did you know that breathing involves both the brain and the lungs? You rarely hear about the critical role your brain plays in monitoring and regulating breathing. Breathing is absolutely essential for our survival; hence it must be under the control of the "higher ups" – your brain. Let's call this the "central respiratory control system."

Your brain is constantly monitoring your oxygen (O_2) and carbon dioxide (CO_2) levels and the ratio between the two. If the O_2-CO_2 levels and their ratio go outside an acceptable range, the brain gives distress signals, or sets off the emergency alarm. When this happens, our thinking brain may also get involved – in modifying, or magnifying the problem – depending on perception, interpretation and other thoughts related to the breathing episode.

Recurrent panic attacks may be defined as a "dysfunction of the central respiratory control system." This happens when the areas of the brain involved in monitoring and protecting the airways from acute respiratory danger (such as suffocation), can become over sensitized and react inappropriately. This dysfunction may be temporary or permanent.

Let's explore the mechanisms of how the central respiratory control system may begin to overreact and trigger an emergency response even though there may not be a real emergency. Here are three popular theories regarding panic attacks and central respiratory control dysfunction.

Brain Suffocation Alarm Theory

The brain is constantly reading oxygen and carbon dioxide levels to protect you from suffocation. When O_2-CO_2 amounts get to unacceptable levels, the brain sounds the emergency alarm. Emergency operation, the body's fight-flight operation, swings into action releasing adrenaline, speeding up heart and lung activity, creating hot flashes, cold chills, and hundreds of other changes that prepare us to either fight the problem or get away from it. This emergency operation, the "fight-flight' reflex, is what we experience in a panic attack.

In addition to checking our breathing and our heart, the brain constantly checks our blood to be sure that we are breathing nontoxic air. If it senses a problem, our brain alarm wants us to run away from the dangerous situation. With COPD, even small changes in the air such as odors, pollutions, pollens, sudden temperature changes, emotional excitement, and hurrying can trigger false suffocation alarms.

Hyperventilation and Hyperinflation Theory

Some people tend to mildly hyperventilate (breathe too fast) often. I call this "over-breathing." Over-breathing can create unacceptable levels of the O_2-CO_2 ratio. When this happens, the body's emergency system takes over, resulting in a panic attack. Over-breathing causes the lungs to hyperinflate, which means that the lungs are not able to get rid of the air they are taking in. (For more on hyperinflation, see chapter March – Week 4: A Look at the Lungs: How are they Supposed to Work and What Went Wrong?) Because the stale air doesn't get out of the lungs, there is very little room for the fresh air to get in. When this happens, you try even harder to take in more air, and as a result, you feel out of breath. You are unable to catch your breath. You become hungry for air. Panic sets in.

Catastrophic Theory

Here we rise beyond the territory of the brain and enter the corridors of the mind. Note that our thoughts, also, can trigger the fight-flight reflex. Theory says that when you think catastrophic thoughts such as, "I may never be able to catch my breath and I'll die" or "I might be having a heart attack and I might not make it to the hospital," such thoughts can signal the brain of an impending danger and set off the body's emergency alarm system.

These theories offer some insight into how body, breath, and mind, interact in a crisis to trigger a panic attack. However, quite often the perceived crisis is not always a real crisis, but an exaggerated view of uncomfortable body sensations made worse by our catastrophic thoughts.

Panic attack symptoms

Experts commonly believe that panic attacks happen due to a highly exaggerated response to these three categories of panic attack symptoms:

1. **Breath-related discomfort**
2. **Uncomfortable bodily sensations**
3. **Catastrophic thoughts**

Here are 13 panic attack symptoms, each in one of the above categories:

1.) Breath-related discomfort

Shortness of breath, smothering
Feeling of choking
Dizziness or lightheadedness, fainting feeling

2.) Uncomfortable bodily sensations

Palpitations, pounding heart, fast heart rate
Chest pain, chest discomfort
Sweating (not due to heat or exertion)
Trembling or shaking (in the extremities or the insides)
Numbness or tingling sensations (parts of the body or the whole body)

Chills, hot flashes (parts of the body or the whole body)
Nausea, abdominal distress
Feeling of unreality or of being detached from self

3.) Catastrophic thoughts

Fear of losing control or going crazy (e.g. "I'm losing my mind!")
Fear of dying (e.g. "I won't make it to the hospital!")

I hope this helps you understand how panic attacks can start and build so next time you will be able to recognize a false alarm and work your way through it, or understand dangerous symptoms and get the treatment you need.

Added Insight

How Can I Tell if its Panic? – a question for Dr. Sharma

Q: How can somebody with COPD or other chronic lung disease know if it is safe to try to relax at home, and "talk themselves down" from a panic episode, or if they are having an exacerbation and should go to an emergency room?

A: First, we must make sure that the person is in continuing care of a physician/pulmonologist, is medically stabilized, and has been educated in the signs of COPD exacerbation: color of sputum, force of coughing, ongoing wheezing, etc., to determine if breathlessness and breathing distress is resulting from the lung condition. If that is the case, call the doctor or go to the hospital emergency room. If that is not the case, then we look at the possibility of a panic attack. Or it could be a third reason, a combination of both panic attack and COPD exacerbation.

In all the three possibilities, we still need to do the following:

1. Calm down our anxiety.
2. Say calming and self-assuring words to ourselves (mental calming or 'talking ourselves down' as you speak).
3. Use pursed-lips breathing (PLB) and make sure we are doing diaphragmatic (abdominal or belly) breathing. (To learn about calming breathing techniques, see chapters July – Week 1 and July – Week 2.)
4. When we have done all that and symptoms have not come under control, we need to call the doctor, or in case of doctor not being available, go to the emergency room.

What we as persons with COPD can do on our end is still the same in all three possibilities. We can use mental calming and correct breathing techniques mentioned above. But when the symptoms continue and don't improve, we call the doctor, 9-1-1, or go to an emergency room. The good news is that the more we learn about panic and anxiety the better we will be able to tell the difference between a panic attack and a medically caused exacerbation.

Ask yourself this:

1. Which of the three theories (Brain Suffocation Alarm, Hyperventilation and Hyperinflation, Catastrophic Thoughts) applies to me?

_____

_____

_____

_____

2. Out of the three "Breath Related Discomforts," which one(s) do I have?

_____

_____

_____

_____

3. Out of the eight "Uncomfortable Bodily Sensations," which one(s) do I have?

_____

_____

_____

_____

4. Out of the two "Catastrophic Thoughts," which one(s) do I have?

_____

_____

_____

_____

Your Turn

Key points, or…if you don't remember anything else from this chapter, remember this:

- Knowing what is physically going on helps in dealing with feelings of panic and anxiety in COPD.
- Your brain constantly monitors your oxygen (O_2) and carbon dioxide (CO_2) levels.
- The brain sets off alarms that are sometimes only false alarms.
- Understanding early symptoms of a panic attack can help you to keep them from taking over and causing a full-blown panic attack.
- It is important to show this chapter and your written answers (below) to your doctor and talk about what specific symptoms you get that indicate the need for immediate medical attention.

Ask yourself this:

Do I have panic symptoms that fit in with what I've learned in this chapter?

This week:

- Remind yourself that not all alarms signal an actual emergency.
- Make a note to discuss this chapter and your above answers with your doctor at your next visit.

March – Week 2

Accentuate the Positive – Every Day is a Gift

"If you expect nothing, you're apt to be surprised. You'll get it."

~ Malcom Forbes

Even if we're doing all the right things: taking our medications, exercising regularly, eating right, and getting enough sleep, there is an all-important element for being pro-active in disease management, and that's maintaining a positive attitude. I'm not saying that our disease is only in our minds. We all know this is not the case. However, I do believe that the mind has a powerful influence over the body, and a negative focus will surely shorten our lives!

We all know COPD can take a terrible toll on us. Each day presents a new set of demands or adjustments. Most of us do learn, eventually, how to live with those physical limitations. But, even if we've modified our activities due to physical limitations, we seem to have an even more difficult time adjusting our mental and emotional outlook. Living with a positive self-image and trying to always look on the bright side can help us heal faster, cope with problems more effectively, and make those required adjustments for a good quality of life.

So, how do we do this? My own approach is simple. *I face each day as a precious gift.* Each new sunrise dawns like a blank canvas. We can paint the day grey, or we may choose the light, bright hues.

The gift of a new day is the best one we can expect to receive. Think about it. It's like getting God's okay to have another go at it. A brand new twenty-four hours – 1,440 minutes you've never ever had before. That's why it's important to unwrap the hours of each day with the anticipation of wonders and joy to be found. Focus on the things you can still do, not on the things you can't. Take pleasure in the small things, find peace and serenity in the goodness that is around us – a child's smile, a mockingbird's song, a neighbor's good deed, time spent with a photo album or journal – all treasures to be found throughout our day.

Does this mean that we should just float through life, thinking only about rainbows and kittens, never giving the day a serious thought? No, not at all. The essence of good emotional health is to maintain a positive attitude while balancing the facts and reality.

Even so, take a moment to review the steps we can take to keep from becoming stuck in the stresses and strains of our limitations. They may seem obvious, but sometimes the simplest things are easy to forget, or taken for granted, so here's a short refresher. Use this as a checklist for your own positive attitude. Look it over – every day if you need to – so you can have more control over your life and greater confidence as you face each day.

- **Keep learning about COPD.** Read articles, attend pulmonary events, and go to reputable websites. The more you know about your disease, the better you will be able to manage it!
- **Follow your doctor's orders.** Develop a good rapport with your pulmonary specialist. Ask questions when you don't understand something or if you disagree with the treatment plan. Know the names of your medications and how they help open up your lungs. Take them as directed.
- **Become part of a breathing support group** – locally and/or online. There is so much we can learn from one another. Go

to meetings. Take in the information. Share your own experiences. Make new friends. Most importantly, give each other support! Only people with COPD can know exactly what you are feeling. Those who don't, including our family members, can only assume.

- **Maintain an exercise routine.** Even a slow and easy exercise program, followed consistently, can help you stay as fit as possible. Do what you can and keep striving to increase it little by little.
- **Smile**. At least five times. Every single day.
- **Be as active as possible.** Fill your life with joy by engaging in activities you love. Enjoy a hobby. Surround yourself with people who care about you, and with whom you can always find something to talk about. Getting out and about takes effort, but we should try to meet that challenge and seek out events and activities that are enjoyable and fulfilling.
- **Don't be too hard on yourself.** You're only human. If smoking caused your COPD, for example, let go of the guilt and shame. What's past is past. You can't change it now and dwelling on it will only drag you down.
- **Keep your sense of humor!** Find a joke or funny cartoon each day, and then share it with somebody. Laugh whenever you can.
- **Focus on what you still** *can* **do**, rather than what you *can't* do.
- **Only you.** Remember that no one else can do these things for you! You, and only you, can breathe for yourself. And you and only you, can choose your attitude.
- **Look at each day as a gift.**

Accentuate the positive, and never underestimate how your upbeat attitude can make a much brighter day for you! Today is a gift. Your gift. Time to open it.

Your Turn

Key points, or…if you don't remember anything else from this chapter, remember this:

- Having a positive attitude can make a difference in not only your emotional, but physical, health.
- You can choose your attitude, even if you have severe COPD.

Ask yourself this:

Have I smiled or laughed today?

This week:

Find at least one positive thing that happens each day this week. Write it in the chart on the next page. On the seventh day look back on your list and see all those good things.

Find at least one positive thing that happens each day this
week, and write it down. On the seventh day look back on
your list and see all those good things.

SUNDAY	
MONDAY	
TUESDAY	
WEDNESDAY	
THURSDAY	
FRIDAY	
SATURDAY	

March – Week 3

Travel with COPD and Oxygen

*"The man who has done nothing but wait for his
ship to come in has already missed the boat."*

~ Anonymous

If you have COPD, travel might seem to be a thing of the past. But it doesn't have to be that way. While a last-minute trip may not be possible, a well-planned one is often doable. Whether you plan to take a car trip with a destination close to home, a flight, or a cruise on the other side of the world, you just may be able to make it happen – if you know how to do it and give yourself plenty of time to plan ahead.

This is by no means a complete list of travel tips for COPD, but it's a start.

Talk with your doctor

The first thing to do is be sure you're healthy enough to travel away from home. Check with your doctor.

Make specific notes outlining the plan you've already made with your doctor about what to do in case of emergency (see chapter October – Week 1: Preventing Exacerbations and When to Call the Doctor).

If you're going away for an extended period of time, say, a month or more, you may need a referral to a pulmonary doctor at your destination. Folks who participate in pulmonary rehab near their seasonal homes are often required by those programs to have a local doctor.

Know the location of the hospital emergency facility closest to your destination. This is just a precaution, and hopefully won't be needed at all.

If you'll be visiting a region with a different altitude and/or climate than you're used to, ask your doctor how it might affect your breathing. Then take the necessary steps to make sure you'll still be able to breathe well.

Medications

Get whatever prescriptions you need for the entire time you'll be gone, with a couple days extra in case of a travel delay (or in case you're too tired to go to the pharmacy when you get back). This should include one for an antibiotic and another for oral prednisone in case of an exacerbation.

If you must fill prescriptions while you travel, working with a nationwide pharmacy (such as Walgreen's or CVS) will make this easier.

Carry copies of your prescriptions with you, as well as a complete list of all the medications you're on: name of medication, dose, and how often you're supposed to take it.

Even if you don't routinely use a rescue inhaler, make sure you have one handy (with spacer or holding chamber). Check to see that it works properly and has enough puffs for eight per day, for as many days as you'll be gone.

Keep your medications and the paperwork with you, within reach, at all times – in a purse, backpack or tote. Don't put them in your checked baggage!

Health insurance

If you have health insurance other than Medicare, check for coverage at your destination.

On your way...

- Keep hand sanitizer handy.
- Drink plenty of water.
- Make sure you have access to handicap (or very close) parking at your destination.
- Arrange for a hotel room that is accessible without stairs.
- Always specify non-smoking accommodations.
- Don't plan two big sight-seeing days in a row. The rest day you have in-between will be well worth it even if you need to miss something.
- Stretch your arms and legs at least every hour or two. This will help avoid painful cramps and life-threatening blood clots! If you're traveling by car, get out and walk around. If you're traveling by plane, train, or bus, get out of your seat and walk up and down the aisle; or at the very least, march in place, lift your legs, or pump your feet on the floor alternating toe, heel, toe, heel, toe, heel.

Oxygen

Life is a bit more complicated if you use supplemental oxygen (We call it supplemental because we *all* need oxygen. You just need a little more.), but don't be scared off by the details of arranging a trip. It is possible!

Start by calling your local oxygen provider, tell them where you're going and ask them what arrangements they can make for you. Ask your pulmonary rehab staff and classmates and/or a COPD online community about what works and what doesn't. Your peers who have traveled with oxygen are a wealth of information and you can learn from their mistakes and their successes.

Unless you're traveling by car, you must call ahead of time (one month is best) to the airline, cruise, train, or bus company, telling them you'll be using your oxygen. Ask them if they require paperwork, such as a doctor's prescription.

Traveling methods

Air – Ask your oxygen provider about renting a portable oxygen concentrator. If they don't have information about it, ask your respiratory therapy professional at pulmonary rehab, and chat with your local or online breathing support group. If you'll be taking a personal oxygen concentrator aboard an airplane, you will need to complete specific paperwork ahead of time. Ask your oxygen company, as well as the airline, what forms you'll need. Your doctor is busy, so allow enough time to have him or her complete and sign the paperwork.

Car – Buckle your oxygen container securely in place with the seatbelt, making sure it doesn't roll around. Make sure your liquid oxygen stays upright and won't tip over on its side.

Ship – As above, you can enjoy a cruise if you use supplemental oxygen. One option is to take a cruise especially for people with chronic lung disease and their guest (see information at the end of this chapter).

Don't give up on getting away!

So many little details…is it worth the trouble? Many folks with COPD will tell you that the trip – and the memories – are well worth it!

Allow yourself time to plan ahead, follow these suggestions, and learn from others who travel with COPD. Then ahhhhh…relax and enjoy your vacation! Don't let COPD cut you off from things that bring you joy. Happy travels!

Your Turn

Key points, or...if you don't remember anything else from this chapter, remember this:

- It takes some extra planning, but travel with COPD and supplemental oxygen is possible!
- Check with your oxygen provider about making arrangements for you.
- Talk with your respiratory therapy health professionals in pulmonary rehab, your local or online breathing support group, about your plans.
- Talk with reliable peers who have traveled successfully – and benefit from their experience.

Ask yourself this:

If I'm not traveling as much as I'd like, is it my COPD that's holding me back?

This week:

If you're thinking about taking a trip, ask your doctor if you're well enough to go.

Here's more help:

The Sea Puffers specialize in group cruises for people with COPD and other chronic lung diseases. www.seapuffers.com

March – Week 4

A Look at the Lungs - How are They Supposed to Work and What Went Wrong?

"If it is to be, it is up to me."

~ Anonymous

This week we're going to take a look at your lungs and how they work. Your lungs are complex, intricately constructed, and delicate – yet powerful and tireless in the performance of their duty. Your amazing lungs are the only internal organ that has direct contact with the environment outside your body. So, as they work, they must take whatever is in the air you breathe and make oxygen available throughout your body, while at the same time, removing carbon dioxide. No matter what insults they encounter, they must be enormously forgiving, continuing to maintain your very breath…and life.

This is a long chapter. But as a COPD educator I know that a big part of learning to live well with COPD is understanding your lungs, how they are made, and how they work. I'm here to tell you – you're smart enough to understand this. We'll just take it one step at a time. If you like, you can read the first two sections, The Lungs from the Outside and the Lungs from the Inside on one day, take a break, and finish the rest of this chapter later.

The lungs from the outside

We're going to learn about the lungs by following the air as it travels through your respiratory system. But before we venture inside the lungs, let's start by looking at them from the outside.

Healthy lungs are nice and pink, soft and spongy, and elastic. Looking at the lungs from the outside, you can't see the bronchi (bronchial airways). These are the tubes in your lungs that the air goes through. This is kind of like when you look at a building from the outside, you don't see all the rooms and hallways, the elevators and passageways, the heating and cooling ducts and all the wires and cables. Yet, you know they're in there, because you know that the building works. The same is with your lungs. Inside that spongy pink tissue, there are many, many tubes through which your air flows, and there are also millions of delicate alveoli (air sacs), and tiny blood vessels that carry the blood which carries the oxygen.

So, here we go. We'll start where the air first enters your body and we'll follow it into your lungs, all the way through the process of respiration.

The lungs from the inside

Upper Airway

Your upper airway includes your nose, mouth, pharynx (the part of the throat behind your nose and mouth), and your larynx (voice box). It might seem overly simple to say that air enters your body through your nose and mouth; although we take that for granted, you must know that the upper airway has three very important jobs to do before the air reaches your lungs. The air must be filtered, humidified, and warmed. If it isn't, the air you breathe will reach your lungs too dirty, too dry, and too cold – irritating your delicate lungs.

The Lungs

Sinus

Pharynx

Larynx

Trachea

Bronchi

Alveoli
cluster

Diaphragm

Bronchiole

Aveoli with
Capillaries

Filtering

The first line of defense for your lungs are the cilia (tiny hair-like structures) in your nose. The cilia help filter out large particles. Have you ever blown your nose after doing a dirty, dusty cleaning or painting project? If you did and saw what was in the tissue, you found all kinds of nasties caught by the hairs in your nose. Good thing that stuff didn't make it into your lungs!

Humidifying

The inside of your upper airway is lined with a thin coating of mucus. The air you breathe is humidified as it passes over this mucus.

Warming

Normal body temperature is around 98.6 degrees Fahrenheit. Unless you're living in the tropics, the air you breathe is not that warm. As the air you breathe passes through your upper airway, it is warmed up.

Bronchi

In a normal adult, about six inches below the larynx (voice box), the trachea (windpipe) divides into two main bronchi (bronchial airways). One leads to the left lung, and the other to the right lung. As your air makes its way through your bronchi, it continues to pass over the mucus, picking up moisture and keeping your airways humidified. Just underneath this thin mucus blanket are more cilia, millions of them, that sweep the mucus upward, trapping dust, bacteria, and other substances (the stuff that made it past the hairs in your nose or mucus in your upper airway). These bronchi progressively branch twenty-two additional times to form more than 100,000 smaller tubes. The tiniest airways in your lungs are called bronchioles.

Alveoli

At the end of each bronchiole are clusters of alveoli (air sacs). Each alveolus is only about 0.3 millimeters (mm) in diameter and just one cell thick – about the same thickness as the wall of a soap bubble or 1/50th the thickness of tissue paper! Normal healthy lungs have more than 300 million alveoli. In fact, if all the airways and air sacs of healthy lungs were laid flat on the ground, they would cover more than 100 square yards. Larger than the size of a tennis court! That's a lot of alveoli, and a lot of surface area to do your lungs' most important job: oxygen exchange.

Oxygen exchange

What is oxygen exchange? Simply, it is the process of getting the oxygen you breathe in, into your blood so it can be pumped by your heart to all areas of your body; and then getting the carbon dioxide out of the blood and back into your lungs so you can breathe it out.

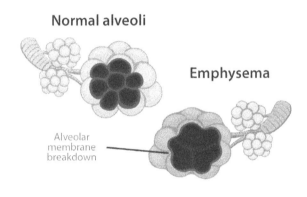

Normal alveoli

Emphysema

Alveolar membrane breakdown

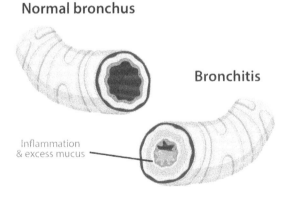

Normal bronchus

Bronchitis

Inflammation & excess mucus

How does this work? Each cluster of alveoli is surrounded by, and in very close contact with, a network of microscopic blood vessels called capillaries. Picture this as a bunch of grapes, with each grape surrounded closely by a fine net. It is here that your oxygen crosses over through the thin walls of the alveoli, and into your blood. After absorbing oxygen, the blood leaves your lungs, is carried to the heart, and then pumped through your body to provide oxygen to the cells of your tissues and organs. As oxygen is used by the cells, carbon dioxide (CO_2), the waste product of this process, is produced. This carbon dioxide is transferred into the blood and carried back to your lungs where it is removed as you exhale (breathe out).

What went wrong? Why is it so hard for me to breathe?

Chronic bronchitis

Let's go back to the beginning. Remember the cilia, the little sweepers in your airways that help keep your lungs clean? Cigarette smoke and other irritants in the environment can destroy or paralyze cilia. This causes them to stop working which means your lungs are not able to clean themselves as they should. Smoking just a few cigarettes, a pipe, or cigar can keep the cilia from working normally. When this happens, your lungs must figure out another way to get rid of excess mucus. This may be why you have a frequent, productive cough.

If mucus comes up with a cough and the cough lasts at least three months for two years in a row, you may have chronic bronchitis.

Emphysema

When lungs become damaged from cigarette smoking or other hazards in your environment, the elastic fibers within them start to break down and come apart. This causes the lungs to lose their elastic recoil, their ability to bounce back after stretching out, making it harder for your lungs to get rid of the stale air. In COPD the "O" stands for obstructive, meaning you have trouble getting the air *out* of your lungs.

Your lung tissue should be stretchy and elastic, like a balloon. The air in a balloon flows out easily because the balloon is elastic (it returns to its beginning shape and size, even after it's been filled up). When lungs lose their elastic recoil, they become more like a paper bag. A paper bag is not stretchy. When air is inside a paper bag, it does not come out easily. It tends to stay there unless it is squeezed out more forcefully. When you cannot get enough air out of your lungs, there is less room to breathe new air in. This leads to a feeling of shortness of breath.

COPD is a combination of chronic bronchitis and emphysema.

Weak airway walls

Another result of loss of the elastic fibers is that the airways lose the strength to stay open. When this happens, they tend to pinch shut or collapse, preventing air from getting out.

Inflammation

Over time, exposure to lung irritants can also cause inflammation (swelling) inside the walls of your airways. When the inside diameter of your airways is smaller than it should be, there is less room for the air to pass through. This makes it harder to breathe.

Bronchoconstriction/ bronchospasm

When your lungs are irritated, the muscles surrounding your airways may squeeze and tighten. This is bronchoconstriction or bronchospasm, causing less air to flow in and out.

Muscles of Breathing

Your main breathing muscle is your diaphragm. It was meant to do most of the work of breathing, pulling down on the bottoms of your lungs so air can flow in easily. When your lungs become over-inflated your diaphragm, which is supposed to be dome-shaped, becomes flatter, putting you – and your lung movement – at a mechanical disadvantage.

But, once again your lungs find a way to compensate. When the diaphragm doesn't work so well, the accessory muscles of breathing are called into action. What is an accessory? It is something that's extra, an add-on. The accessory muscles are around your collarbone, your neck, and between your ribs. The problem with using accessory muscles is that they weren't meant to do all the work. They aren't able do a great job of moving your air. Using these muscles to breathe not only takes a lot of energy but it can cause your shoulders and back to become tense, sore, and tired. More work of breathing plus less efficient lung movement adds up to a whole lot of effort without a lot of results. No wonder it's so hard to breathe! (For more about the muscles of breathing, see chapter July – Week 2.)

I know some of this is hard to hear. Your amazing lungs, designed to do their job so well, so miraculously, are permanently damaged. It's normal – and it's alright to be upset when you first learn this. But once you start coping with this reality, you can settle down and get the information you need to move on and do your best to breathe better every day.

Added Insight

Oxygen transport and obstructive vs. restrictive lung disease

How much oxygen is in our air?

The mix of gases that make up the atmosphere here on earth

contains about 78% nitrogen and 21% oxygen. The remaining one percent is made up of argon, carbon dioxide, water vapor, and other trace gases.

Hemoglobin and oxygen transport

If you've ever watched a freight train go by, you know there are many types of train cars: coal cars, tankers, automobile carriers, boxcars, and more. Coal, for example, can travel only in a coal car. No matter how much coal has been mined and is ready for transport, if that train doesn't have enough coal cars, there will not be enough coal being carried and delivered.

It's the same with oxygen. Oxygen can latch onto, and be carried by, only one type of blood cell – the red blood cell or hemoglobin. Even if your lungs have enough oxygen, this oxygen can't get where it needs to go if there is not enough hemoglobin. This is one of the many reasons it's important to maintain a healthy red blood cell count and not be anemic.

Obstructive vs. restrictive

COPD is an *obstructive lung disease*, a combination of emphysema and chronic bronchitis. Obstructive lung disease means you have *trouble getting the air out*. This obstruction can be caused by mucus in the airways, airways that tend to collapse easily, or airways that are narrow due to inflammation (swelling) or constriction (tightening). People with obstructive disease cannot easily exhale all of their air, leaving some air in the lungs at the end of exhalation.

In *restrictive disease*: pulmonary fibrosis, interstitial lung disease, asbestosis, sarcoidosis, etc., the lungs are scarred and stiff. This is more of a *problem getting the air in*. It can prevent full expansion of the lungs as well as make it harder for oxygen to cross over from the alveoli into the blood.

Your Turn

Key points, or…if you don't remember anything else from this chapter, remember this:

- It is important to know how healthy lungs work and what goes wrong when you have COPD.
- You have the right to know this, and you should know this even if it's hard to hear.
- When you know what's going on inside your lungs, you can do a better job taking care of your breathing and doing what you can to stay as healthy and active as possible.

Ask yourself this:

Do I have a question about how the lungs work? If so, jot it down and ask your doctor, respiratory therapist, or other lung health professional about it.

This week:

See chapters July – Week 1 and July – Week 2 for helpful breathing techniques. If you're ready to learn even more, see chapter July – Week 5 to learn about different types of breathing medications and how each one works on specific problems in your lungs.

Here's more help:

www.copdfoundation.org

March – Week 5

Compassion, Renewal, and Rediscovery with COPD

"The will of God will not take you where the grace of God cannot keep you."

~ Anonymous

Do you ever take the time to reflect on how living with COPD has affected you? I don't mean the loss of things we can no longer do because of our physical restrictions. I'm talking about the way we look at ourselves and others that may have changed.

It's funny how, when we are faced with illness and/or disability, life has a way of teaching us some very good lessons, whether we want them or not. We learn the value of life, and how we should never take it for granted. We learn that life is fragile, and that we – all of us – are mortal.

Compassion

I think that, for me, one of the most lasting things I have learned from living with chronic disease is compassion. In the ten years since I've been diagnosed with COPD, I have changed. I am less judgmental. I can empathize with those who also endure a serious illness or disease. My heart goes out to a person with a disability of any kind. I'm more willing to lend a helping hand or a sympathetic ear to others who are ill, especially those with lung disease. I like to think of it as a patient developing more patience. And I believe this all translates into compassion.

I've learned, too, that through the involvement with my support group I have found great joy in helping other COPD patients. And I know that in helping others, it gives me back so much more than I give – even the power to heal – if not my body, my spirit.

Being mindful of other people's feelings and needs helps us become less centered on our problems – and it certainly makes us easier to be around! It opens doors to new understanding and helps bring peace to our own state of mind. Just think of the good you can do by opening those doors; the help you can bring, the comfort you can give to others. And when we help others, we help ourselves as well.

What about you? Has having COPD caused you to become more sensitive in dealing with others? Has it helped you to be gentler and more caring? Has it made you better able to understand someone else's challenges? Has it made you more grateful, more patient, more compassionate?

Renewal

We might say that as people with COPD we have been given a bad sentence, dealt a difficult hand to play. Yet, we have more reasons than just about anyone to seek emotional growth and acceptance, and to do it with grace. Learning to do this leads to renewal. This involves finding aspects of ourselves that were always there, allowing us to feel content – even under the stress of chronic disease – and to feel joy with others or simply with ourselves.

Throughout the coping process that comes with any chronic disease, we confront terror, loss, rage – all kinds of emotional pain. But when we are able to face both the loss of what we had in the past, and fear of the unknown, we're on our way to achieving some level of renewal. In finding this strength and facing the dreads of disease we learn that living with this disease is not so overwhelming after all.

Renewal is like finding ourselves again. This is our same self but in new circumstances; yes, with constraints to handle, but with the tools to forge on regardless of changes and loss of the ability to do things we once loved.

Renewal is not passive. It is a changing attitude towards our relationship with COPD, born of all our past struggles. Each day brings new challenges, and through this, we learn to set and reset our priorities in such a way that the limitations of our disease no longer define us.

Rediscovery

I am my same self, but in a new set of circumstances. Simply, I'm the same me – but a me with COPD.

Instead of focusing on what our disease makes us, it can become more a matter of "Who do we *choose* to be, given our limitations?" Yes, we have a choice! It is entirely possible to be physically disabled, or we may call it "challenged," or "limited," without being emotionally handicapped.

We can separate ourselves from the fact that we have this disease, COPD, and be creative about adapting, and focusing on pleasure and the things we still *can* do, rather than on our limitations and things we *cannot* do. We should do our best, also, to use some of our energy to help other people and remain actively involved with living.

We shouldn't judge ourselves too harshly. We should live our lives with few regrets, then give ourselves credit for the effort it takes. We must forgive ourselves for what may have happened in the past and focus on the joys of rediscovering what makes us unique. When we do this, we'll be able to accept our disease, along with the positive changes that can come when we find ourselves living with COPD.

Appreciate the compassion to care more about others and embrace the renewal of realizing that we're still the persons we were.

With this, we can take better care of ourselves and rediscover finding joy in things we can still do.

Your Turn

Key points, or…if you don't remember anything else from this chapter, remember this:

- Having COPD can help you to become more understanding, patient, and compassionate.
- You're not a different person because you have COPD. You're still you.
- You are more than your disease.

Ask yourself this:

- How have I changed, as a person, since being diagnosed with COPD?
- Do I ever feel like I've lost the "old" me?
- Am I able to separate my COPD from the person I am inside?

This week:

- If you feel that you are more compassionate, do something kind for a person who is in need of understanding or help.
- If you're struggling with feeling like the "you" you always were, write your feelings down and/or find someone to talk with about it. A counselor who specializes in people with chronic disease is best.

April – Week 1

Could You Have Alpha-1?

*"If you do not ask yourself what it is you know, you will
go on listening to others and change will not come."*

~ Saint Bartholemew

It was Mary Pierce's fortieth birthday. As she stood in the kitchen her phone rang. It was not a call from a friend to wish her well, but it was her doctor with news for Mary that would change her life.

"I was right," he said. You have this thing called Alpha-1 Antitrypsin Deficiency. It's inherited."

For years Mary had been struggling with shortness of breath, repeated lung infections, severe, unexplained weight loss, and a major decrease in tolerance for physical activity. All along the way she blamed herself.

"When I started getting symptoms, mainly the weight loss and shortness of breath, I thought, "You dummy, you've got to stop this. No doctor's going to be able to do anything for you until you quit smoking."

She flashed back to the time when a friend came to visit from California. It was this friend's idea to go play tennis. After running for just three balls Mary was in trouble. I thought, "Hey, what's going on here? I can't breathe!"

But at that point she could not admit to herself she had a breathing problem, let alone admit it to her friend. "I faked it and said, 'It's really too hot. Let's not play.'"

Mary's reason for not playing tennis that day was the first in a long line of excuses she made for why she could not do what healthy people usually find easy. Over the next ten years she tried to quit smoking. She took several stop smoking classes, and although she had cut down to around a half a pack per day, she continued to smoke. But her breathing wasn't getting any better. Mary's weight continued to drop, and she hid her increasing shortness of breath from family, friends, and co-workers, doing everything possible to pretend she was okay.

"I've got to quit smoking. Nothing's going to happen until I stop smoking. I'm a good Catholic girl. I took all the guilt on myself. I said to myself, 'Don't expect anybody else to help. I've got to do it my own dumb self. My smoking is doing it.' So that's how I rationalized it."

Mary's dad had died of emphysema and her mom of lung cancer and emphysema. Her husband's father had also died of lung cancer and emphysema. Both Mary's parents had smoked cigarettes. When aunts and uncles came over to play cards the house was full of cigarette smoke. She started smoking at about age 13, sneaking cigarettes.

You might think that it was, indeed, *all her fault*. Not so. What Mary didn't know at the time was that she had a genetically inherited disorder causing her lungs to lack protection from cigarette smoke and other environmental irritants. The damage was occurring at an accelerated pace and far more destructive than it would have been to a person how didn't have Alpha-1. At age thirty Mary had the lungs of an old woman.

"Then one time I was all weekend sitting up in a chair, struggling to breathe, really struggling. I thought, 'Man, if I have to live like this I don't want to live anymore.' Monday morning came and I called the doctor. At that point I weighed 99 pounds. He took one look at me and said, 'You're too young to have this much lung disease.'"

Back to where our story began…the doctor continued, "You have this thing called Alpha-1 Antitrypsin Deficiency. It's inherited. They're doing some experimental treatment at the NIH (National Institutes of Health). We can try to get you into a clinical trial."

"That gave me some hope," said Mary. "Then he added, 'They're also beginning to do lung transplants.'"

"Transplants! That's the one thing that told me how bad it was." (At this point in time there had been only one lung transplant done on an Alpha-1 patient in all of North America.)

"I can remember myself standing in the kitchen, hanging the phone up, and saying to myself, 'OK, what do we do now? What do we do to make this go away?'"

Over the following months, in spite of doing all she could to maintain her breathing and her health, Mary's lung function declined to a meager 14% (30% is considered severe, 25%, disabled). She was on oxygen full time and had just ordered a wheelchair when she received a phone call that would again change the course of her life.

But this time it was good news. The transplant coordinator at the University of Michigan said they had lungs for Mary. Lung transplant, for any lung disease, is extremely complex. After an uneventful transplant surgery, followed by an unusually successful post-transplant course, Mary is still doing well today.

Over twenty years after that fateful phone call, Alpha-1 Antitrypsin Deficiency is still hugely under diagnosed. Awareness is abysmal, even among many physicians and those in the health care community. Patients with Alpha-1 see, on average, several doctors over the course of several years before being correctly diagnosed. They are often told they have severe asthma or that they have severe COPD at a young age caused by nothing but cigarette smoking. The vast majority of people with Alpha-1 do not receive transplants and must live with advanced COPD at an early age.

In spite of progress with increased awareness, dedicated research, and better treatments, we still have a long, long way to go. Finding Alphas early in the course of their disease empowers them to seek the best treatment and stay as healthy and strong as possible. If you have COPD you should know about this genetic disease and ask yourself, "Could I have Alpha-1?"

Alpha-1 facts

- Alpha-1 Antitrypsin Deficiency (Alpha-1) is a condition that is passed from parents to their children through their genes.
- This condition may result in serious lung and/or liver disease at various ages.
- People with Alpha-1 have received two defective alpha-1 antitrypsin genes: one from their mother and one from their father.
- Alpha-1 occurs when there is a lack of a protein in the blood called Alpha-1 antitrypsin or AAT.
- The main function of AAT is to protect the lungs from inflammation caused by infection and inhaled irritants such as tobacco smoke.
- Alpha-1 Antitrypsin Deficiency (A-1AD) is one of the most common serious genetic conditions in the U.S. and is more common than cystic fibrosis.
- The World Health Organization (WHO) has recommended that all individuals with COPD, and adults and adolescents with asthma, should be tested for Alpha-1.
- Alpha-1 can cause liver disease in children or severe liver and lung disease in adults, most often causing early emphysema.

- It is estimated that 100,000 people in the U.S. have Alpha-1.
- Alpha-1 diagnosis is often missed, even by doctors.

Source: Alpha-1 Foundation www.Alpha1.org

Added Insight

John Walsh's story
In memory of Helen Chase Walsh

In the Dutch Colonial home on Cheviot Street, life was very good. Robin Hood Road circled the neighborhood, with its sparkling lakes and beautiful woods. Helen Walsh, a former high school home economics teacher, was married to Jack, a popular high school football coach and college scout. The two had met years before while teaching at the same high school. Everybody loved Jack; gregarious, positive and generous. And everybody loved Helen. It seems as if it would be a wonderful life for her, and it was – living in the beautiful Northeast countryside, with a loving husband, four bright, beautiful children, and adoring friends. But there was something very, very wrong with Helen Walsh. She couldn't breathe.

Two of her children were twin boys, John and Fred. Fred recalls, "I remember her being skinny, struggling, her nose was running all the time, but she never once complained. Never. Ever. She was hiding what she was going through each and every day. I think back now and realize that she never went up the stairs with me. She always went ahead or behind, because when she got to the top, she couldn't catch her breath."

John says, "She never let us know just how sick she was. I mean, we knew she couldn't get out of bed, and she had the O2 [oxygen] on. But we never thought she'd die."

Helen Chase Walsh died at age forty-six in 1963, the same year her mysterious killer was identified in a medical research lab in Sweden.

It was Alpha-1 Antitrypsin Deficiency.

"Fred and I were diagnosed with asthma and we talked with each other. I had a bout of pneumonia; he had a couple bouts of pneumonia. We were getting sick more frequently. It was obvious to us that our 'asthma' was really making us sicker than we thought asthma should. Freddy was very diligent about getting a more thorough diagnosis and pursued that."

John continues. "So, Freddy called me up, let's see, right around our fortieth birthday and said, 'I've got good news and bad news.' Being the eternal optimist, I said, 'Give me the good news.'

"He said, 'I know what we have. A genetic condition called Alpha-1 Antitrypsin Deficiency.'

"I said, 'Alpha-what?' He explained what it was—and that it... was genetic. And I said, 'I know what the bad news is.'

"Yeah, that's what Mom had."

"And here we were at forty years old. Mom died at forty-six. We kind of looked at each other over the phone and said to each other, 'There's just no way we want to progress as rapidly as Mom did, and there's no way we want our children to go through losing a parent.'

"We made a commitment to each other right then that we were going to find out everything there was to know about Alpha-1, and we were going to do whatever we could to avoid the foreshortened life, and do whatever necessary to figure out what we needed to do, health-wise.'

"So we went in and asked, 'What's our life span?'

"'We don't know,' they said."

"Should we move to Arizona or Florida?"   "'We don't know.'"

"This was 1989, twenty-six years since Mom died and since they discovered Alpha-1! Freddy got frustrated and said, 'What's the oldest person you actually know with Alpha-1, doctor?' "

'We really don't know...well...we... had someone who came in here last week who was 50.'

"It was very obvious to us then, what they didn't know. I mean, this was the Mecca for health.

They explained, 'We can't solve everybody's problems. Unless you organize the investigators, unless you organize the community, unless you raise money and work with us and put pressure on us to do the research, it's not gonna get done.'

"And then I knew. I knew what I had to do. In January 1995 we founded the Alpha-1 Foundation. It was a huge risk. But we were doing the right thing. My dad always said, 'If you don't feel the arrows hitting your back, you're not leading.'

"Mom exemplified the spirit of someone who doesn't want to give up, who wants to have a good quality of life, who doesn't want anybody to feel sorry for them. You know, it isn't, 'The glass is half empty. The glass is half full.' I'm hearing everybody saying, 'We've got to fix this.' And I can't think of doing anything more meaningful."

In his work with Alpha-1 John Walsh discovered an even bigger and largely unrecognized community; those with COPD. He went on to become the founder of the COPD Foundation which he led for over twelve years. John passed away on March 7, 2017 as a result of complications from an accident in 2016. He was sixty-eight years old. He is greatly missed.

Your Turn

Key points, or…if you don't remember anything else from this chapter, remember this:

- Alpha-1 Antitrypsin Deficiency (A-1AD) is one of the most common serious genetic conditions in the U.S. and is more common than cystic fibrosis.
- Alpha-1 is often misdiagnosed as asthma or common COPD

due to smoking.

- Testing for Alpha-1 is done with a simple blood test.
- Members of a vibrant Alpha-1 community are ready and willing to help Alphas breathe better and live full lives.

Ask yourself this:
Could I have Alpha-1?

- Are you age 20-50 and short of breath with little effort?
- Did you quit smoking with no improvement?
- Do you have frequent lung infections?
- Do you have asthma, emphysema, chronic bronchitis, or bronchiectasis?
- Do you have a family history of lung disease?
- Do you have cirrhosis of the liver with no history of alcohol?

This week:

If you answer "yes" to any of these questions, talk with your doctor about getting tested.

Here's more help:

www.alphaone.org – Alpha-One Foundation 877-228-7321

April – Week 2

How to be Able-Hearted When You Can't be Able-Bodied

*"No one is useless in this world who light-
ens the burdens of another."*

~ Charles Dickens

As people with COPD, we go through many changes in the progress of our disease. Shortness of breath and fatigue often lead to more limitations and less tolerance for exercise, so we need to adapt. Over time, these limitations result in a loss of the ability to do many things we used to do.

COPD is a chronic disease, one that won't go away, and it has no cure (at least for now). All this could cause a terrible loss of self-esteem and independence for us, which could result in just giving up and withdrawing from the rest of the world, and feeling sorry for ourselves, expecting people to do everything for us. It could – but it doesn't have to.

So, how do we make it through this defeatism? Well, we learn to make adjustments in our lives and follow our COPD management plan every day. Moreover, we accept ourselves as we are, doing what we're able to do while knowing our limitations. And we must do this without holding on to the anger or bitterness we may have felt when we were first diagnosed.

The very process of evolving to a healthy emotional state can be daunting. Being emotionally healthy means we must not judge ourselves, comparing what we do now to our previous physical capabilities. Our bodies may be less able than they were in the past, but our minds are not!

So, here it is – the good news you've been waiting for! Even if we're not able-bodied, we can still be "able-hearted." We can discover in ourselves something beyond physical constraints and learn to help others. It might take some creativity, but it can be done. Working from the inside out, we can find ways to live a full and productive life by helping others; knowing that even if what we do seems insignificant, it can have a positive effect on that person, and it can be very rewarding for us.

If you have COPD, even if it is advanced, you can still be useful. Your work on Earth is not done. You can help others and discover the reward of knowing you made a difference.

Here are some ways you can be "able-hearted:"

- Accept yourself as you are now, even though you might not be able to do what you once did.
- Focus on today, not yesterday or tomorrow.
- Learn to ask for help – and accept it – when needed. Without shame.
- Maintain social contacts with friends and family.
- Take a creative approach to the use of your limited energy.
- Keep a sense of humor and fun.
- Help others. Here are thirteen things (some that take little or no energy) you can do to help someone; and there are hundreds more you can do. Remember, some of these actions might seem like nothing at all, but they make a difference – more than you know.

- » Smile at someone.
- » Say "thank you" with a smile and eye contact.
- » Tell somebody, "You look nice today."
- » Write a thank you note.
- » Call a friend to wish them a good day.
- » Read to a child.
- » Listen to a child read.
- » Pray for a friend in need.
- » Pray for world peace.
- » If you're able, make cookies for somebody who deserves a treat.
- » Make baby hats or blankets for your local birthing center.
- » Do a small repair project for a friend or neighbor.
- » Be compassionate (maybe that person is worse off than you are).

Do your best to take tomorrow in stride, whatever it may bring. Be confident that each day will provide opportunities for positive experiences. Expect good things. Don't let the good stuff slip by because you have become entangled in a web of hopelessness and despair.

Forgive yourself for what you can no longer do. Celebrate the things you *can* do! Search deep inside for the strength – and the heart – to live graciously and with caring. Live each day with no regrets…for things as they are now, not for things as they might have been. Allow yourself to peacefully coexist with your COPD.

The ability to be connected to ourselves, to others, and to the world around us far outweighs the physical limitations we have. Remember, you are not just a person with COPD. You are more than that, and you are able-hearted!

Added Insight

Jeanette's story

Long before it was common to hear of cultural diversity, my Aunt Jenny routinely opened her home to people from many different lands. I have vivid memories of her, her daughter, and my mother busily serving Sunday dinners at my aunt's home. The table was so overloaded with food, that there was a tea cart in the doorway to the kitchen, next to my aunt's chair bearing more food.

As a young child, squeezed between my father and my sister, I'd sit at that table across from my Native American cousin, her husband of Dutch descent, and their children. Between bites of baked potato and roast beef, I'd learn something from a special guest about life in Sweden, Arabia, Germany, Peru, Switzerland, India, or some other faraway place. But most importantly, I learned that people are people – good people – no matter where they come from. At the close of the meal our guest would offer a prayer in his or her native tongue. Nobody but our guest understood the words, but I knew that God did, and that just made everything feel all right.

Jeanette grew up on her family's small farm twenty miles south of downtown Chicago in the time of The Great Depression. The oldest of three children, she spent much of her time working in the onion and tomato fields. "I had to wear those big bib overalls and they were hot! My sister and brother and I spent many hours pulling tomato worms off each plant. We put them in a bag and then burned them. Those were the days before pesticides. There was no irrigation and every evening we'd go out with buckets of water to give each plant a drink."

When not doing chores or attending school, Jeanette taught herself to read music at home by playing an old pump organ with the only written music they had, a hymnbook. In the days when most young women didn't think of going on to education beyond the eighth grade, let alone high school, Jeanette attended college on a scholarship, majored in pre-law, and pursued vocal training in Chicago. Following college, she worked as a legal assistant in a small, smoked-filled office for just short of fifty years. She never smoked cigarettes herself.

She and her husband, Art, traveled overseas and shared their home throughout the years with many people from around the world, including missionaries, foreign exchange students, and youths who needed guidance. They became foster parents to a Native American girl whom they eventually adopted. Jeanette's parents had told her, "Work hard and share what you have."

She began to notice difficulty breathing after she contracted tuberculosis while visiting with a missionary at a tuberculosis hospital in Arabia. Ten years later she was diagnosed with COPD. In spite of severe COPD, she believed that keeping a positive attitude and staying busy within limitations, helped her live each day to the fullest with her lung disease.

Not long before she died, I asked her, "If you could say one thing to somebody with COPD, or any chronic lung disease, who is about to give up, what would you say?"

Without hesitation she replied, "Do something to help someone. Some things you cannot do, but there are many things you can."

Your Turn

Key points, or…if you don't remember anything else from this chapter, remember this:

- Even though your physical abilities may have changed, you are still useful and valued.
- Accept yourself as you are.
- In helping someone else, you help yourself.

Ask yourself this:

What can I do to help somebody today?

This week:

Do at least one thing on the "ways you can be able-hearted" list.

April – Week 3

Nutrition

"Don't dig your grave with your own knife and fork."

~ English Proverb

Disclaimer: Always consult your doctor or a registered dietician (RD) before making changes to what you eat. This is not intended as medical advice.

They say, "You are what you eat." It's easy to see why that makes sense when you're trying to lose weight, gain weight, or if you have issues with your heart or your digestive system. But, does what we eat have any effect on our breathing? And if so, how? In this chapter we'll look at some basic guidelines as well as questions about proper nutrition with COPD.

Good nutrition is important for everyone, and it's especially important if you have COPD. Food is the fuel your body needs to perform all activities – including breathing. Good nutrition helps the body fight infections, the very infections that can settle in your lungs and lead to pneumonia. For the person with COPD, shortness of breath can make eating difficult just when you need to eat well to maintain your health and strength. This week we'll explore ways to eat right and maximize your food intake to produce energy and stay healthy and well.

Your body uses food for energy as part of a process called metabolism.

Metabolism: Food + Oxygen = Energy + Carbon Dioxide

In the process of metabolism, food and oxygen are changed into energy and carbon dioxide.

Food provides your body with nutrients (carbohydrates, fats, and protein) that affect how much energy you have and how much carbon dioxide is produced. Energy is needed to not only perform activities of daily living, including sleeping, but to simply keep your body alive. Carbon dioxide is a waste product that leaves your body when you breathe out.

It's important to maintain a healthy body weight. Ask your healthcare provider or registered dietitian what your "goal" weight should be, and how many calories you should consume per day for optimum health.

If you are overweight, your heart and lungs must work harder, making breathing more difficult. In addition, the extra weight might demand more oxygen. To achieve your ideal body weight, exercise regularly and limit your total daily calories. If you are overweight, dropping just 10% of your weight will make it easier to breathe and take stress off your knees and back.

Conversely, being underweight is a serious problem for many people with COPD. This is addressed below.

Here are some commonly asked questions about nutrition and COPD. You'll note that some of the foods recommended as good to eat might also be found on another list of foods to avoid. Not everybody can tolerate every food, so pay attention to what you eat and how it affects you and adjust your food plan accordingly.

1.) What should I eat to breathe better?

Eat a well-balanced diet of protein, carbohydrates, fruits, vegetables, and yes, even fats. Eat lean meats, whole grains rather than white bread and rice, and healthy fats such as olive oil. Eat the rainbow – foods with a variety of colors – bright colors (candy doesn't count!). These are foods such as tomatoes, dark leafy greens, carrots, broccoli, squash, red peppers, and citrus. If you have a large grocery or farmer's market near you, consider trying one new fruit or vegetable each week. Eating a variety of foods from all the food groups will provide the nutrients you need.

2.) Are there foods I should avoid, foods that make it harder for me to breathe?

Avoid foods that cause gas or bloating. A full stomach or bloated abdomen can push up on your diaphragm (the main muscle of breathing) and make breathing difficult. Not all foods listed below cause everyone to have gas or bloating. Pay attention to what you eat and if it causes problems for you, avoid it and see if you begin to feel better.

Foods that are more likely to cause gas and bloating include:

- Carbonated beverages
- Fried, greasy, or heavily spiced foods
- Beans, broccoli, Brussels sprouts, cabbage, cauliflower, corn, cucumbers, leeks, lentils, onions, peas, peppers, radishes, scallions, shallots, and soybeans.

Don't waste your energy eating foods that provide little or no nutritional value (such as potato chips, candy bars, colas, and other snack foods). Avoid eating more than one or two pieces of candy per day.

3.) Why do I get so tired when I eat?

You might be eating too fast, you might be hunched over, or you might be talking while eating. If your doctor has prescribed supplemental oxygen, you might not be wearing your oxygen as you should. If you become exhausted while eating, here are some tips that may help:

- Take your time.
- Chew slowly.
- Put your fork down after every few bites.
- Sit up straight in a chair with good back support.
- Use pursed-lips breathing.
- Choose foods that are easy to prepare so you still have energy for eating.
- Ask a family member or friend to help with meal preparation.
- Check to see if you are eligible to receive Meals on Wheels.
- Freeze extra portions of what you cook so you have a meal already prepared when you're especially tired.
- Rest before eating so you can enjoy your meal.
- Try eating your main meal earlier in the day so you have enough energy to last the day.
- Wear your oxygen while eating.

For tips on saving energy in the kitchen see May – Week 2: Making the Most of the Breath you Have – Energy Conservation and Work Simplification.

4.) Why do I feel so full after a meal and find it even harder to breathe?

Over-inflated lungs, often the case in COPD, can press down on the stomach. In turn, a stomach that is distended with food or gas pushes up and compresses the lungs. No wonder it's hard to breathe! Eating frequent, small meals, up to six per day, will take up less room in your stomach, can help you feel more comfortable, and put less stress on your system.

5.) Do dairy products cause me to produce more mucus?

It depends on the person. Some people find that milk and other dairy products tend to either increase the amount of mucus or make it thicker. If this is your concern, try reducing dairy products. After doing this, if you find that the amount of your mucus and/or the thickness is reduced, talk to your doctor or a registered dietician about it.

If you eat dairy products, and it does not seem to make your mucus worse, then it's alright to go ahead and eat them. Again, pay close attention to what you eat, see how it affects you, and if you find that a certain food causes a problem for you, talk with your doctor or a registered dietician about avoiding it.

6.) I'm shrinking! How can I gain weight?

Did you know that the simple act of breathing takes more energy for people with COPD? A person with COPD may need an extra 430-720 calories per day, just to do the work of breathing! If you have COPD it's important for you to take in enough calories to produce energy in order to prevent weakening of the diaphragm and other muscles. Your body needs fuel and if you've run out of fat, your body will begin to burn muscle. Don't burn your breathing muscles for fuel!

Keep in mind that a poor appetite may be due to depression, which can be treated. Your appetite is likely to improve after depression is treated. Ask your doctor about this.

If you're at or below ideal body weight and have COPD, check with a registered dietician about starting a weight gain plan. He or she may recommend you take a nutritional supplement in addition to healthy, high-calorie meals.

Here are a few ideas for snacks to help you put on or maintain your weight:

- Pudding made with whole milk
- Soft or semi-soft cheeses
- Granola bars
- Custard
- Tortilla chips topped with melted cheese
- Crackers with peanut butter
- Bagels with cream cheese – not reduced fat cream cheese
- Cereal with half and half
- Fruit or vegetables with dips
- Yogurt with granola
- Dried fruits
- Premium ice cream
- Cookies and brownies
- Popcorn with margarine and parmesan cheese
- Breadsticks with cheese sauce

7.) What's the best beverage to drink when you have COPD?

As much as some of us love our coffee (or our wine!), we must remember that good old water is the best thing we can drink for our health. You should drink at least six to eight eight-ounce glasses of non-caffeinated beverages each day, to keep mucus thin and easier to cough up. If you need to get up at night to urinate, drink more of these earlier in the day to avoid extra trips to the bathroom during the night. If you're trying to gain weight, check with a registered dietician about the best beverages for you.

8.) What about salt/sodium and retaining fluid?

We just talked about the importance of drinking fluids, but some people with COPD who also have heart problems, may need to limit their fluids.

If you have a problem with swollen feet and legs, it may be due to extra fluid in your body, forcing your heart and kidneys to work harder. One way to keep from retaining fluid is to decrease your intake of sodium, or salt. It is generally recommended that we consume no more than 1,500 milligrams (mg) of sodium per day, and less, if you have fluid retention as mentioned above.

It's possible to eat well with a reduced sodium diet. Here are some tips:

- Use herbs or no-salt spices to flavor your food.
- Don't add salt to foods when cooking.
- Keep the saltshaker off your table.
- Read food labels and avoid foods with more than 300 mg sodium/serving.
- Use a salt substitute approved by a registered dietician. There are many choices available.

Monitoring your weight every day is recommended. If you are taking corticosteroids to reduce inflammation, your weight may fluctuate significantly. If you have an unexplained weight gain or loss (two pounds in one day or five pounds in one week), contact your doctor. If you take diuretics (water pills), you might also need to increase your potassium intake. Check with your doctor. Some foods high in potassium include oranges, bananas, potatoes, asparagus, and tomatoes.

9.) What about vitamins and supplements?

Most balanced diets contain enough vitamins to meet your basic needs. On the other hand, taking a multi-vitamin is safe and may be helpful. Ladies, check with your doctor if you should be taking added calcium for strong bones.

Be aware that some diet supplements can interfere with your prescription medications or even cause health problems. Always check with your doctor before taking something, even if it is a non-prescription over the counter (OTC) product.

10.) What about fiber?

Include high-fiber foods such as vegetables, cooked dried peas and beans, whole-grain foods, bran, cereals, pasta, rice, and fresh fruit in your diet. Fiber helps move food along the digestive tract and control blood glucose levels. A good goal is to consume 20 to 35 grams of fiber every day. Here's an example: 1 cup of all-bran cereal for breakfast, a sandwich with two slices of whole-grain bread and 1 medium apple for lunch, and 1 cup of peas, dried beans, or lentils at dinner.

Good food plus oxygen is the fuel we need for energy – and for living! Modifying your eating habits will not cure COPD, but it can help you feel better.

Show this chapter to a registered dietitian and ask what you can do to eat for your best possible health. A RD can give you safe, detailed, nutrition guidance and help develop a personal action plan for your optimal nutrition.

Your Turn

Key points, or…if you don't remember anything else from this chapter, remember this:

- Eating right for COPD can help you feel better and breathe better.
- It is harder on your breathing if you are overweight; and underweight is also a challenge.
- If you have COPD, it is not safe for you to be under what is considered your "ideal" body weight.

Ask yourself this:

Am I doing all I can to eat right with COPD?

This week:

Staying within any restrictions or special nutritional guidelines given to you by your doctor, make at least one change in your nutrition and/or eating habits.

April – Week 4

Coping with Stress

"Don't hurry, don't worry. You're only here for a short visit so be sure to stop and smell the flowers."

~ Walter Hagen

Life with any chronic disease has its share of stress – those of us living with COPD are prime examples of that. COPD results in major compromises to our lifestyles and activities. We may lose our independence, suffer from periodic bouts of depression, even tend to isolate ourselves from friends and family – all the time fighting for our breath! We may feel anxious, nervous, or overwhelmed. Yes, indeed, I would say that stress is a regular visitor to those of us with COPD.

What does it take to get through this stress? What works for one person may not work for the next. We all need to find the coping skills that work best to bring us out from under the dark clouds, back to clear, blue skies. I hope you have some of your own stress-relieving methods. Here are a few of mine. Maybe they will help.

Meditation

A few minutes of quiet solitude can provide me with a chance to meditate my way free (at least, temporarily) of emotional – and sometimes physical – stress and strain. I focus on my breathing, taking deep breaths in and slowly exhaling until my mind becomes clear of all the things that have been pulling at me. Then I guide my thoughts and visualize a soothing, peaceful scene. Sometimes it's by the ocean on a warm, sunny day where I can smell the salt air and hear the waves. Other times it's a serene Irish garden by a pond, and I can imagine smelling the roses and freesia as I hear birds singing in the trees. I have many other favorite places to "go" (with visualization) in times of stress. Fifteen minutes of meditation like this brings me comfort and assurance that I will be alright.

T'ai chi Ch'uan

This ancient Oriental form of stretching seems to help me drop the weight of worries, especially those caused by COPD. It is a gentle form of exercise that even people with COPD can learn and do, and it helps keep my body toned and limber. I practice it a couple of times a week, more if I need it. I recommend tai chi as a wonderful muscle conditioner, even if you aren't able to engage in a strenuous exercise routine.

Music

Soft, classical music has a calming effect on most people, but whatever works for you is best. I enjoy taking a few minutes with my feet up, listening to quiet classics. I have one that has classical music set to the sounds of the ocean – truly the best of all sounds for my ears! Just a few minutes away from the worries of the day brings me peace and contentment.

Games

If I need a super-strong distraction from stress, I can play against the computer in a game of Scrabble. I'm not brave enough to play real people online, although it can be done. Doing this totally distracts me from obsessing about problems I can't do anything about. A game takes about twenty minutes and I don't have to look for someone who wants to play.

Exercise

There's nothing like a good walk outdoors (on breathable days) to get rid of the cobwebs in my brain and relieve the stress of COPD. If you can't walk, try exercises designed to help your breathing muscles or to help condition your whole body. Exercise is one of the best stress busters!

Journaling

I recommend this for everyone! You'd be amazed at how much better you feel, and how much the load will have lightened after you've expressed your feelings by writing in your own private journal. For your eyes only, this journal should be off limits to anyone else. And, oh yes, feel free to write in your journal on the good days, too. It doesn't have to be reserved for just the negative feelings.

As the song goes, "These are a few of my favorite things..." to help me over the humps of bad days, stress, and worries. One more thing – it helps to remind myself that the current bout of stress won't last. It makes it easier to know I can work my way through it, rather than let it take me over and control my entire existence. Whatever it is that is bothering me, it doesn't deserve that kind of importance in my life! Or in yours!

My solutions may not be right for you. The important thing is to be aware of the many coping skills available to help us conquer the stress of life with COPD. Make your own list of favorite things and keep them handy for those days when you're stressed out from dealing with COPD.

Your Turn

Key points, or…if you don't remember anything else from this chapter, remember this:

- It is normal to feel stress when you have COPD.
- There are many things you can do to control stress.
- It's a good idea to have more than one way to handle your stress.

Ask yourself this:

Do I have a method for controlling my stress that works for me? (Cigarette smoking doesn't count!)

This week:

When you feel stressed, try one of the stress-reducing methods described in this chapter.

May – Week 1

The Emotional Impact of Being Diagnosed and Living with COPD

"A man who says he has never been scared is either lying or else he's never been any place or done anything."

~ Louis L'Amour

Do you remember the day you were diagnosed with COPD? Many people do. Although you may have seen it coming, it still hits hard to hear the doctor say, "You've got COPD. It is a progressive disease and there is no cure."

If you think back to when you were first diagnosed, your thoughts at that moment may have been swirling with shock, regret, confusion, sadness, anger, and a hundred questions. You may have felt that your whole life was in a state of upset. You may have felt, or still feel, as if your future, the plans you made, were gone forever – that your life, as you knew it, had been taken away from you.

When you have been diagnosed with COPD, help most likely begins with medically-related changes: new medications, possibly oxygen, among other things. But in addition to these therapies, it's essential that you also learn about coping emotionally with the disease and with the changes taking place in your life.

The "Take Back Your Life" framework may help. In the column on your left you will see some "Issues:" common feelings, emotions, and emotional issues related to being diagnosed, and living, with COPD. Note that this is not a list of stages with one following after another. You could easily be experiencing more than one issue at a time. And just because you have worked your way through an issue, that doesn't mean you will never have it again. However, it's important to know that if that happens, it certainly doesn't mean that you have failed.

The "Pathways" are in the middle column and involve ways to help work through each issue. These are called "Pathways" rather than "solutions" or "answers" because they may come in different forms and may take a while – maybe a long while – to work through. It takes some time to walk a path, you may see and experience different things along the way, and you may even stumble. But you know that as long as you stay on the path, you're more likely to find your way to where you want to go.

In the right-hand column, the "I Get It – and I'm Going to Be Okay!" is how you might feel or what you might say after you've made your way along the "Pathway," the process of understanding and coping with the "Issue." Reaching the "I Get It" doesn't mean you're an expert in coping. It means, simply, that you recognize the problem, you understand it, and have found your way to dealing with it effectively in an emotionally healthy way.

Take a look at the "Take Back Your Life" framework on the next two pages. Where are you?

"TAKE BACK YOUR LIFE" FRAMEWORK

© Jane M. Martin 2020

The Issue	The Pathway	I Get It! (and I'm going to be okay)
Denial I don't have COPD or emphysema. I was fine until I got that last cold. This is just bronchitis.	**Recognition** Recognize the fact that you have COPD.	I may not like it, but I guess I do have this COPD thing, and at least now I know what I'm dealing with.
Fear Knowing I have COPD scares me. A lot. But I've always been a strong person so I can't let anybody know how frightening this is for me.	**Validation** Realize that it's okay – and normal – to be scared about this diagnosis.	I'm not weak. It makes sense for me – or anybody who has COPD – to be fearful at first. My feelings are normal.
Loneliness I'm all alone. I must be the only one who has this. If there are others, where are they?	**Voice** It is estimated that 30 million people in the U.S. and 210 million worldwide have COPD. There is strength in numbers and those numbers are beginning to be heard.	I am not alone! There are millions of others out there with the same, or similar, concerns.

"TAKE BACK YOUR LIFE" FRAMEWORK

© Jane M. Martin 2020

The Issue	The Pathway	I Get It! (and I'm going to be okay)
Confusion Inhalers, nebulizers, oxygen... this is just too much to take in. I'm constantly confused and overwhelmed, and my breathing is out of control.	**Education** Learn all you can about COPD from solid, credible sources. Ask your doctor to refer you to pulmonary rehabilitation.	Now that I understand what's going on in my lungs, how to take my medications, and work my equipment, I know what I can do to make my breathing as easy as possible. I'm in control of what I do.
Isolation Nobody understands what I'm going through. They can't possibly know what it's like to be so short of breath.	**Support** Join a local breathing support group, pulmonary rehabilitation, online support group, or all of these.	It really helps to talk to, and be around, others with the same problem. They under-stand.
Despair I'm useless. I can't do anything anyore. I'm of no good to anyone.	**Service** Do something to help someone, a person with or without COPD.	There are things I can no longer do, but there are many things I can do! My friends, my family, and my community need me. My life has meaning again!

Added Insight

Helping ourselves – a question for Dr. Sharma

Q: What is the best thing we can do for our emotional well-being in our everyday life? How can we keep from getting discouraged, or at least deal with it better? How do we prevent our illness from taking over our life?

A: Emotional work, like any other part of self-care or medical care, requires us to constantly work on it, like you take medication "A" three times a day, medication "B" twice a day and an inhaler as soon as you notice something coming on. Emotional work is never complete. You just keep getting better at it if you keep working at it.

So, surround yourself with positive people, books, quotations, affirmations, visualizations, pictures, and objects. But above all, remind yourself that you must spend as much time as possible keeping a positive mental attitude. Don't focus on what you have lost, but on what is left. Find a positive meaning for your life and your disease.

When you experience troubling symptoms, see yourself getting past them and getting better. Keep a calm attitude by telling yourself something like, "If I get more angry, frustrated, anxious, or depressed, it won't be helpful. If I stay positive and somehow manage to put a smile on my face or find something funny to laugh about, I will be helping the healing forces."

These are just a few thoughts for a start. Yes, there is something right in the age old saying, "mind over matter."

Your Turn

Key points, or…if you don't remember anything else from this chapter, remember this:

- Being diagnosed with COPD will most likely change your life.
- For most people, coping well with the diagnosis and life with COPD is a process and does not come all at once, but gradually over time.
- It is possible to work through the emotional issues and enjoy a full and happy life with COPD.

Ask yourself this:

Where am I on the "Take Back Your Life" framework? Remember, you might be on more than one "Issue."

This week:

If you are in the "Issue" column in any of the six steps, try starting out on your pathway. If you are in any of the "I Get It!" boxes, good for you! Go down the chart and see how you're doing on the other issues.

Here's more help:

COPD 360social online community. www.COPDFoundation.org

May – Week 2

Make the Most of the Breath You Have - Energy Conservation and Work Simplification

Rivers know this: There is no hurry. We shall get there someday.

~ A. A. Milne

Probably one of the most common concerns in pulmonary rehabilitation is expressed in this way: "I can do a lot here. I'm walking for twenty minutes on the treadmill, I'm working with weights and everything. Why do I still get short of breath when I'm walking out to my car?"

No matter how well somebody does in pulmonary rehab or exercising on their own, even though they're making progress by increasing their walking distance and improving their endurance, strength, and flexibility, if it doesn't make a positive difference in their everyday life outside the gym, we've somehow missed the mark.

Learning energy conservation and work simplification tips and techniques forms a bridge from gym to home. It can help you benefit from the gains you make in physical fitness and make a huge difference in the way you live, improving your quality of life on a day-to-day basis.

Below are some of the basic concepts of energy conservation and work simplification for people with COPD. Working with a certified occupational therapist can maximize your ability to do what you need – and want – to do in your everyday life, with as little shortness of breath as possible.

Pace yourself

Pacing is one of the most important things to learn. In pulmonary rehab when patients talk about what causes them an increase in shortness of breath, something that often comes up is "rushing" or "hurrying." When you have COPD with significant shortness of breath, you simply cannot rush or hurry. Instead, you can learn to move at a slower, but steady pace while using correct breathing techniques.

Listen to your body

There will be days when you wake up and know almost immediately that it's going to be a "bad air" day and there's no use in denying it. Take it easy that day and don't feel guilty about it! (See chapter February – Week 3: Good Days, Bad Days.) Or you may wake up feeling great and up to a special task that you have been saving for a good day. The important thing is to learn to listen to your body, trust your instincts, and go with them.

Breathe right

Using correct breathing techniques can go a long way in helping you feel less short of breath. When you are performing any kind of activity, always exhale during the hardest part, blowing your air out as you lift, bend, or climb stairs. If you are short of breath, stop and rest for a minute before resuming your activity.

Even if you don't go to pulmonary rehab (and I hope you do!) you can still benefit from learning simple, common sense techniques. Some of these are actions that once you've learned them, you'll wonder why you never thought of them before. You know, just because you've always done something a certain way, doesn't mean it's a good idea to keep on doing it that way – especially if you're limited by shortness of breath!

Once you get used to taking a fresh look at how you do everyday tasks in order to save energy, you'll be on your way to better breathing. Here are a few tips and techniques to save your energy. Note that these are just suggestions. It's best to work with a certified occupational therapist.

Avoid unnecessary activities

Ask yourself, "Is it really necessary that I do this? What will happen if I don't? Can it wait?" Avoid unnecessary activities that cause you to expend more energy. For example, wear a terry cloth robe after your bath or shower to save yourself the effort of drying off. Allow the dishes to air dry instead of drying them by hand, or better yet, use the dishwasher. Sit, don't stand, to do your hair, shave, or put on your makeup. According to the Canadian Lung Association, sitting uses 25% less energy than standing. Or, if you can't sit, at least prop your arms up when doing your hair, make-up, or shaving.

Organize your activities

Plan your most strenuous activities at the time of day when you have the most energy. Alternate between tasks that are difficult, and those that are easy. Plan out rest periods and don't feel badly if you need more rest on one day than another.

Organize your closets, shelves, and drawers

Place items you use most often between waist and shoulder height. This way you won't have to do a lot of bending or stretching to reach them. Keep all items in the area in which you use them to avoid taking extra steps to find them. For example, store living room cleaning products in a basket in or near the living room. Saving steps saves energy.

Run a fan

If you are bothered by the heat or feel confined because of stale, stagnant air, use a small portable fan. A portable fan is useful in any room. It will help you cool off, blow offensive or irritating odors away from you, and give you the feeling of moving air.

Maintain good posture

If you move your body properly, you will save energy. Avoid excess bending or lifting. Use better body mechanics when trying to move items by pushing, pulling, or sliding them. Instead of carrying things, get yourself a little wagon or cart to wheel them.

Carry heavier loads close to the center of your body

Carrying an oxygen tank or heavy purse over one shoulder can cause pain and fatigue, even shoulder injury. When possible, carry items such as this on a strap that goes across your chest or back, using the core of your body to carry the load. Ladies, we all love our handy handbags, but stop and ask yourself, "Do I really need to have all this stuff with me?" Maybe you can get by with simply a money and credit card/driver's license clip, tissue, inhaler, and lipstick in a cute little bag that hangs across your body and rests on your hip. Keys can be clipped to the outside if they're too bulky to go inside.

Practice relaxation

When you relax, you help restore energy to your body. Make sure to schedule relaxation periods during your day and when doing so, concentrate on relaxing all your muscles and slowing down your breathing.

Wait to do activities an hour or more after eating

Digestion draws blood with its oxygen, away from arm and leg muscles, leaving them less able to move for extra demands. You may find you feel your best soon after taking your medication or having a breathing treatment.

When you have COPD, try looking at it as a matter of supply and demand. Think of your supply of energy in the same way that you think of money in the bank. There's only so much of it and it must be spent wisely. Repeated "overspending" can cause a deficit in your breath. And we all know what happens when we spend more than we have!

Learning energy conservation and work simplification tips and techniques can make a big difference in the way you live, improving your quality of life so you spend less time huffing and puffing, and more time enjoying life.

Added Insight I

Climbing stairs

Disclaimer: Always consult your health care provider before starting any new activity. Show this to your doctor or respiratory health profession-al and ask him or her if it would be appropriate for you. This is not intended as medical advice.

One of the most common problems I hear from people coming into pulmonary rehab is that they become extremely short of breath when climbing stairs. Here's a suggested method, but don't try this for the first time when you're alone.

- Hold firmly onto the handrail.
- Relax your shoulders and take a nice breath in through your nose. Blow your air out slowly through pursed lips, twice as long as you breathed in (see chapter July – Week 1 on pursed-lips breathing).
- Still holding onto the stair rail, take another nice breath in through your nose. Start climbing the stairs only as you exhale, and while slowly and gently blowing your air out through pursed lips. Let's say you inhale (breathe in) for a count of two. Then, try to exhale (breathe out) for a count of four. In this case, climb just four steps.
- Stop. Do not let go of the handrail.
- Breathe in again through your nose for a count of two.
- Breathe out through pursed lips for a count of four, climbing four more steps.
- Repeat. (If you breathe in rather than exhale as you climb, you will tend to hold your breath and that can make your shortness of breath even worse.)

By using this technique, it may take a little longer to go up those stairs, but you'll reach the top with breath to spare!

Added Insight II

In the kitchen

Food preparation and clean-up can be a big drain on energy and breath. Here are some tips for breathing easier in the kitchen.

- Don't try to do everything at once. Set smaller goals. Almost all jobs can be divided into segments.

- Plan your meals when you are neither hungry nor tired. Don't waste your time and breath on unhealthy foods. Every bite counts.
- Use convenience foods when you have to but remember that many packaged foods have high salt and sugar contents. Learn to read labels.
- If you enjoy cooking, make double or triple the amount of your favorites when you're feeling good. Freeze them and enjoy tasty, easy meals when you need a day off.
- Microwave ovens and slow cookers make food prep easier and reduce heat in your kitchen.
- When cooking, always use your exhaust fan, or make sure there is good ventilation.
- Keep your most used pots and pans on top of the stove. They're heavy, and you're going to use them again anyway! Consider doing the same for dishes and flatware that you use often.

Your Turn

Key points, or…if you don't remember anything else from this chapter, remember this:

You can save energy – and breath – if you learn some tips and tricks of energy conservation and work simplification.

Ask yourself this:

What are three things I find the most difficult to do?

This week:

If possible, apply what you've learned in this chapter to save energy on those three things. If you don't know how to do this, ask your doctor for a referral to an occupational therapist. Remind your doctor that this will help you remain more independent, and possibly even help you avoid acute exacerbations.

Here's more help:

For more energy conservation tips specifically for eating, see April – Week 3: *Nutrition*.

For more energy conservation tips specifically for attending holiday parties, see December – Week 2: *Nine Ways to Help you Breathe Better and Save Energy this Holiday Season*.

May - Week 3

Gardening and Yardwork

To our friends in the southern hemisphere, this week, read chapter September – Week 3: Facing Fall – Preventing Exacerbations and When to Call the Doctor.

"To be surrounded by beautiful things has much influence upon the human creature; to make beautiful things has more."

~ Charlotte Perkins Gilman

When new patients arrive at pulmonary rehabilitation on the first day, I ask them about their goals, "What do you hope to improve or change as a result of coming to pulmonary rehab?" Without a doubt, one of the most common goals is the ability to get outside again to enjoy some gardening.

For those unfamiliar with COPD, this might seem simple, but when you struggle to breathe in the first place, getting outside in the warm weather, moving around, bending over and lifting, can seem impossible. So, how can you, a person with COPD, still work in your yard or garden with energy enough left over to enjoy it?

A true story

Leona, a patient in our pulmonary rehab program came in one day really disappointed – and actually quite peeved. She said, "Tammy, my daughter, told me my gardening days are over. Done! She won't let me do it anymore. She says I get too out of breath. That makes me so mad!"

"Oh my," I said. "I know Tammy's just trying to help. She worries about you." I paused. "Hmmmm...I'm sure you can still to do *something* – you just need to know how – pace yourself and breathe the right way as you do it. We'll figure it out."

So, I researched, found some great information and gave it to Leona. "Show this to Tammy when you see her on Sunday and let me know how it goes."

We'll get back to the story of Leona and Tammy in a minute, but first, here are some tips on gardening with COPD. Some of this might take a little planning and a bit of an investment, but it'll be worth it if it means you can work in your yard and still have the energy – and the breath – to enjoy it!

Plantings

- Reduce the total size of your gardening area and flower beds, focusing on your most favorite plants.
- If you become breathless by getting on the ground and bending over, consider replacing the ground-level areas of your garden with easier-to-reach raised beds.
- Trade your traditional garden for window boxes.
- Decorate your deck, patio, or terrace with container gardens.
- Use perennials that come up year after year without replanting.
- If you have a large yard, consider replacing some of your

garden or grass areas with low-maintenance ground covers or no-maintenance stones or wood chips.

Tools and equipment

- A nylon garden hose, fifty feet long with its reel, weighs only 2 1/2 pounds and can be carried in one hand.
- Use lightweight tools that require less energy: for instance, trade in your traditional hoe and rake for smaller versions with extra-long or extendable handles.
- Use a long-handled gripper for removing gardening debris from the ground.
- Keep tools together in a rolling cart to avoid taking extra steps back to get them from where they are stored. If you are able to carry them, keep them in a lightweight bucket or basket.
- If bending over cuts off your breath, try sitting down to work. You can do this with containers and using a lightweight folding stool or a rolling cart with storage and a sturdy seat.

Weather and the air

- Listen to your local weather report, or the Weather Channel or other source on television or online. Avoid working outside when allergen, pollen, and pollutant levels are high.
- Limit your exposure to intense heat and humidity; garden during the cooler times of the day, early morning and late afternoon.
- Know if you are allergic to things growing in your garden and lawn. If you are and don't want to give up your gardening, use a dust mask while you work.

As you go

- Cut down weeds while they are still small and leave them where they fall. It makes good mulch.
- If possible, relocate your garden tools and hose closer to your garden.
- Garden in moderation – especially in the spring when you're raking and preparing beds. Do a little at a time.
- Ask for help – whether it's carrying trays of annuals, bags of dirt, or weighty annuals, have someone else do the heavy lifting for you. This includes getting your purchases into and out of your car. A young person in your neighborhood may be able to help.
- Gently stretch and warm your muscles before and after you do your gardening.
- Slow down, relax, and alternate cardio-intensive activities (i.e., reaching, walking) with tasks requiring less exertion.
- Incorporate frequent breaks into your routine to reduce fatigue.
- If you mow your grass, wear a dust mask. Better yet, have a family member cut the grass, hire someone to mow the lawn, or trade in your walking mower for a riding mower.
- For small lawns, if you're able, use a push-mower rather than being exposed to the fumes of a gas mower.

Raising monarch butterflies

This is something popular with folks in our pulmonary re-hab program. If you can find milkweed, you will probably find Monarch Butterfly eggs if you know how to look. Caring for and raising a Monarch is easy, fascinating and fun! Look online for more information.

For the birds

If you've always enjoyed feeding the birds but it has become too much for you, you can still keep a birdbath. Position the bath near a hose, preferably one with a high-pressure nozzle. All you need do is spray it with high pressure to keep it clean and make sure it's filled. Thirsty birds will still stop in and you can enjoy watching them splash and drink.

So, what ever happened with Leona? I'm happy to report that two weeks later she came into rehab, beaming. "Tammy stopped by yesterday with a bunch of flowers. We're going to plant them in some pots out on the deck. I'll have my garden after all!"

Leona's garden might be smaller, it might be different, but it's still something she can work on and enjoy the beauty of nature outdoors.

Remember to pace yourself, think creatively, and ask for help when you need it. Happy gardening!

Your Turn

Key points, or…if you don't remember anything else from this chapter, remember this:

- You can still have a garden, even if you have COPD.
- If you use just one or two tips or techniques, it could make a big difference in helping you continue with the yard work and gardening you enjoy.

Ask yourself this:

Is there a tip or technique in this chapter I can use to make my gardening easier?

This week:

Review this chapter and commit to making three changes that will make your gardening or yardwork easier, or your time outdoors less work and more enjoyable this year.

May – Week 4

Exercise

What saves a man is to take a step. Then another step.

~ Antoine de Saint-Exupery

Disclaimer: Always consult your health care provider before starting an exercise program. The following are basic suggestions for those who have been approved to do exercise and are under the supervision of a doctor or pulmonary rehabilitation professional. This is not intended as medical advice.

If you have COPD and are short of breath, it's a good possibility that the last thing you want to do is exercise. But, of all the treatments for COPD, exercise might just be the one thing that can make the biggest difference in the way you move, the way you view your disease, even the way you look at life.

Being a respiratory therapist working in pulmonary rehab for many years, of course I would love to see every person with COPD go to pulmonary rehab to learn how to exercise safely in a monitored environment. Unfortunately, that's not possible, so here are some exercise basics for your information. Show this chapter to your doctor and ask if it would be okay for you to start an exercise routine.

Types of exercise

Stretching and flexibility exercises help improve your posture, movement, and breathing. Stretching the right way can reduce or even eliminate muscle soreness brought on by exercise. Flexibility activities can reduce your chance of falls or other injuries.

Strengthening and resistance exercises help build muscles, improve strength, and maintain bone health. Lifting hand weights, using resistance bands, and working with weight machines are good ways to increase your strength.

Endurance and aerobic exercises help improve the function of your lungs and heart. Walking, biking, rowing, stepping, and swimming, are just a few endurance exercises. When done correctly, this type of training builds stamina and endurance with shortness of breath you can control.

Breathing techniques

Always use pursed-lips breathing during exertion of any kind, but especially with exercise. Using correct breathing techniques will help you do more while feeling less short of breath. When you are lifting weights, exhale (blow your air out) as you lift. Never hold your breath! Always keep your shoulders relaxed and use the diaphragmatic (abdominal or belly) breathing technique, if possible. If you become short of breath, stop and rest for a moment before starting again. See chapters July – Week 1 and July – Week 2 for pursed-lips and diaphragmatic breathing.

Getting ready

- Dress comfortably in clothes that move with you. Wear

supportive shoes that fasten snugly, and socks that cushion your feet and absorb perspiration.

- If you have a fast-acting Beta-2 agonist (rescue medication) inhaler, ask your doctor if you may use it fifteen minutes before the start of exercise to maximize the openness of your bronchial airways.

- If your doctor has recommended that you use supplemental oxygen during exertion, ask your O_2 provider to set you up with a portable, lightweight system. Make sure you know how long it will last!

- Start slowly, even if you feel you can do more. If you have not exercised in a while you need to give your body a chance to get used to it again. Don't overdo it on the first day! A muscle that may not hurt today might tell you loud and clear tomorrow that you overdid it! In some programs exercise time is increased by one minute each session (under the direction of an exercise specialist) unless a person is able to do more.

- After stretching, begin with a three-minute warm-up. This means go slow and easy for the first three minutes. Don't go full out on cold muscles.

- Do cool down stretches as directed by an exercise specialist. Stretch just until you feel a gentle pull. Don't bounce!

- Let's say you want to walk outside, and you know you're able to walk for ten minutes non-stop. In this case you should walk for five minutes, then turn around, and go back to your starting point. Check out your walking route ahead of time (by driving your car) to see if there are any places to sit down or lean on if you need to take a break. Don't get stuck somewhere out there with no breath left to get you home!

- If it's okay with your doctor or physical therapist, add weight or resistance training to your routine. Lifting soup cans or bottled water can help you increase your strength.

- Don't exercise on an empty stomach. Have a light meal or a snack before your work out. Carbohydrates and protein work well. If it is approved for your diet, peanut butter or cheese on crackers or a peanut butter sandwich is good. Add some fresh fruit and eight ounces of water and you're ready to go!
- If possible, exercise in a group or with a buddy. It will keep you motivated, be more enjoyable, and make sure help is there if you need it. If you must exercise alone inside, keep it interesting! Exercise where you can look out a window, watch TV or listen to peppy music. If you walk outside alone, walk in the daylight and carry a mobile phone.
- If you're in a pulmonary rehab program you'll be monitored by the staff to make sure your oxygen, heart rate, and blood pressure are at safe levels. If exercising on your own, you can monitor your oxygen saturation and heart rate, if you have been trained by a specialist in pulmonary exercise on how to work out safely.

Check to see if you qualify to participate in pulmonary rehab. Even if you're significantly short of breath and don't think you're able to exercise, you might be surprised at how much you can do. Pulmonary rehab is a great way to learn safe and appropriate exercise and tips to keep you breathing easier.

Added Insight

Should I exercise when I'm sick? – a question for Helen Sorenson

Q: I've been ill a lot in the past six months. (congestion, fever, coughing, SOB). Every time I'm sick, I seem to lose everything I gained through exercise. Is there anything I can do when I'm ill to avoid losing what I accomplished exercising when well?

A: When you are sick you usually don't have the energy or the desire to exercise. I will tell you that lying flat in bed will cause you to lose muscle mass much quicker than if you are sitting up. Just by sitting up you are putting tension on the muscles and bones and you will not lose as much strength. So, when you are sick, get someone to help you sit up in bed, or in a chair during the day. If you need it, wrap yourself in a blanket with a box of tissues, bottle of water, oxygen, applesauce, nutritional drinks, and anything (TV remote, music, find-the-word puzzles) to keep you occupied. Just sitting up will help prevent loss of strength, so when you get over the acute phase of the illness, you will not have so much ground to make up.

I know I don't feel much like eating when I am sick, but that is also very important. Good nutrition will help strengthen your immune system and help you get better faster.

If someone (grandkids, a friend, a good neighbor) will help you move your arms and legs, a form of passive exercise, it will increase blood circulation to the muscles and also help prevent loss of strength.

Your Turn

Key points, or…if you don't remember anything else from this chapter, remember this:

- People with COPD, even very severe COPD, can and should exercise.
- Exercise improves strength, flexibility, and endurance – and also helps with circulation and feelings of well-being.
- Do pursed-lips breathing with any exertion, but especially during exercise.
- Check with your doctor before starting any exercise routine.

Ask yourself this:

Am I exercising regularly? If not, why not? What's keeping me from it?

This week:

- If you are already involved in routine exercise, ask yourself if it's time to increase your workout time and/or intensity.
- If you're not, ask your doctor about starting a pulmonary rehab program.

Here's more help:

- To find a pulmonary rehabilitation program near you, contact the American Association for Cardiovascular and Pulmonary Rehabilitation http://www.aacvpr.org. Phone: (312) 321-5146.
- Call your community senior center (even if you're not a senior) for information on low level exercise classes, television shows, or videos.

June – Week 1

What Can I Count on Today?

"Better to lose count while naming your blessings than to lose your blessings while counting your troubles."

~ *Maltbie D. Babcock*

With twinkling eyes and a happy smile, Josie was a favorite patient of mine. She carried herself with confidence and grace – yet a bit of mischief – in spite of severe COPD and having suffered loss and betrayal in her past.

"So, how do you stay so cheerful, in spite of your bad lungs – and everything else?" I asked.

"It's simple, darling. I ask myself every morning, 'What can I count on *today*?'" Josie uttered the word, "today," in a hushed, almost reverent, tone. I looked at her, puzzled. She told me a story. And I'm sharing it with you here.

It was four o'clock on a hot summer afternoon in 1962. Josie, a single mom, punched the clock at the aircraft factory, jumped in her car and picked up her girls. Her modest wage covered rent, food, clothing, and fuel for her car, but little more. So, although Josie wasn't able to take her girls out to movies or buy them many toys, with a spark of creativity and a flare for adventure, she gave them a good life. And today she had a special surprise she was sure her girls, Patty age seven, and Connie age five, would love.

"Let's go girls! We're off to the lake to go swimming!"

The girls were thrilled! That afternoon the three had a great time, playing in the water and swimming until they headed home after seven p.m.

The next day, same as always, Josie picked her girls up after work. "Girls, I have another surprise for you today. We're going for ice cream!"

The girls were not nearly as thrilled at the thought of this as they were with swimming the day before. But on they went to the ice cream shop. Josie reached into her purse for the last of her meager change, just enough to pay for three scoops of ice cream in three waffle cones. The mom and her daughters climbed into the car, eating their treats and heading for home.

Patty and Connie sat low in the back seat, sulking. They looked at each other and began to chant, "We want to swim! We want to swim!"

"Girls…"

"We – want – to – swim!" they said, more loudly each time. And they kept it up.

Josie said, "Give me your cones."

The girls continued to fuss. "We – want – to – swim!" the chant went on.

"Give me your cones!"

Quiet now – and a bit confused – they handed their mother their ice cream cones.

With her left hand on the wheel, and her right hand holding two half-eaten ice cream cones, with one swift stroke Josie tossed the cones out the driver's side window.

"Mom! Our ice cream! Why'd you do that?" The girls began to cry.

"Yesterday we swam, and we had a wonderful time. Today we

can't go swimming. You had a nice treat in your hands but all you could do is complain that it's not what you had yesterday. Forget yesterday and appreciate what you have today."

People with COPD learn very quickly that life is worth celebrating. As chronically sick people, we seem to appreciate life more, probably because we realize that good days are precious and the time we have left may be brief.

Still, even if we have been living with COPD for a long time, we may need to be reminded of the joy of just living; even having a sense of wonder for what each new day will hold. Who can tell if this day will provide us with special memories to file away for later recall? What if this is the day when we get a chance to do a good deed for someone in need? What if this is the start of improved health for me? Who knows? This might be the day that a cure is found for emphysema; when research finally proves that lung tissue *can* be regenerated. Or, more simply, how about I just enjoy my favorite meal this evening?

There are so many ways we can celebrate life. Each of us should have our own list of favorite things to do. Sure, a great time for me might be less than exciting for someone else. But we all know what special experiences bring a lift to our heart, a little dance to our step.

One thing we can all do to help us celebrate life, is find ways to help others. There is great joy to be found in spreading good will. Maybe we can choose a day to bring lunch to one of our fellow COPD'ers who has been confined to home. Or perhaps we can just bake some cookies for a favorite person, or as a way to say a special thank you.

It could be that someone you know would appreciate help with picking up a grocery item. Or maybe you can drop off a copy of a good book for someone else to enjoy. The list is endless. And it is easy enough to find activities that don't require a lot of physical exertion.

Try to accept each day with the grace of a life well lived. Make the most of its opportunities. Fill the blanks and voids of your daily existence with positive thoughts and events.

I look back on the prognosis I was given fifteen years ago – two to five years – and I am grateful that I am still alive, still able to contribute to life around me, and still able to function in my daily business of living.

Quality of life for people living with any chronic disease may be hard to find sometimes, but it is possible! People with COPD learn that life is worth celebrating, and that each new day dawns with a whole new world of reasons to enjoy it.

Your Turn

Key points, or…if you don't remember anything else from this chapter, remember this:

- People with COPD often learn to appreciate each day more so than those who are well.
- Finding joy in each day enhances quality of life.

Ask yourself this:

What can I count on today?

This week:

Find an activity each day that gives you joy in that moment and write it down in the chart on the next page. On the seventh day look back on your list and see all those good things.

Find an activity each day that gives you joy in that moment
and write it down. On the seventh day look back on
your list and see all those good things.

SUNDAY	
MONDAY	
TUESDAY	
WEDNESDAY	
THURSDAY	
FRIDAY	
SATURDAY	

June – Week 2
Dying with COPD

"The question is not whether we will die, but how we will live."

~ Joan Borysenko

"What will it be like when I die? Will I just struggle for every breath and gasp until I can't get any more air? That sounds like a horrible way to go! That's what scares me the most."

As a respiratory therapist I've heard concerned, frightened – and rightfully so – COPD patients ask these questions and express their fears many times. I don't have all the answers, not by a long shot, but I am here to tell you this: The answer is "No." If you are an informed patient, dying, whether you have COPD or not, does not have to be about pain and suffering. Rather, it should be all about care and comfort, along with dignity and personal choice. Your dignity. Your choice.

Let's talk about a subject none of us – whether or not we have COPD, no matter how old or young we are – really want to talk about. Our final days of life.

Never say die?

It's important to tell you that my patients in pulmonary rehab are generally the kind of folks who pretty much never say die. They are spunky and spirited even when things get tough. However, many of them do get to the point at some time or another when they say, "You know what? I'm just tired. I gave it all I had. I far outlived what the doctors said I would. And I am totally at peace with leaving this life."

If you have "end stage" (I hate that term), or very severe COPD with significant shortness of breath, you might be asking, "Is this it? Am I at the end of the road?" Many times patients have come into our program on the first day, thinking for sure that this was "it" – and once they got started in rehab they found there were many things they could do to breathe better and live longer, some of them living many years longer than anybody had predicted.

Is this the "end of the road?"

As you ask the "Is this it?" question, you must ask yourself these questions too:

- Do I have a good doctor who takes time with me and listens to what I have to say?
- Have my doctor and I discussed, and ruled out, all treatments for my COPD, including lung transplant and other surgery or procedures?
- Am I on solid, maximum treatment for COPD; best practice medications, and oxygen if my tests indicate I need it?
- Have I discussed taking medications such as prednisone that would help me breathe better even if they might have some unwanted long-term side effects?
- Do I exercise regularly, even if very slow and minimal?
- Do I have a support group; family, friends, and other people with COPD who understand what I'm going through?
- Do I find it difficult to feel happy anymore?
- Have I had tests or screening to rule out any other major problems, such as heart disease?

If you answered yes to each of these questions, and you've done all you can to keep going, every step is a struggle, nothing relieves your shortness of breath, and you find it hard to feel joy in life, it is a good time to have a talk about this with your doctor.

What if this is "it?" Here are a few thoughts on dying with COPD.

Hospice care

First of all, it's important to understand that calling hospice doesn't mean you have one foot in the grave and the other on a banana peel! It's alright to be in hospice, even when you're still active! In fact, sometimes it even can allow you to be more active than you've recently been. People involved in pulmonary rehab can be enrolled in hospice and still come to maintenance (self-pay) exercise class.

Being in hospice takes pressure off of you, wondering how you're doing, and if you're doing the right things. And it takes a lot of stress off your loved ones. It bears repeating, it is alright to call hospice. Just think of it this way – if you talk with the people from hospice and they say you don't qualify, wouldn't that be good news?

Put it in writing

Complete an advance directive. There are two parts to this: designation of an advocate who would speak for you if you were ever unable to speak for yourself; and a living will outlining the care and treatment you want and the care and treatment you don't want. Everybody should have an advance directive, even if they're young and healthy. For more on advance directives, see chapter October – Week 2.

Share your story

Everybody has a story to tell, and we should all pass ours along, whatever our age or health status. Make plans for a friend or a grand-child to listen as you tell your story while recording on audio, video, or digitally. Just sit down and start talking. You'll be so glad you did! Then, someday, even after you're gone, your words – and your spirit – will live on, bringing joy to your loved ones.

Spend time together

Make sure your family and friends understand that although a loved one seems to be "out of it," or unconscious, very often they can still hear. A dying person can hear who is in the room, the news of the day – "Grandpa, I hit a home run today!" – and most importantly, those precious "I love you's" right up to the end.

Give permission

If you're the loved one of a person with COPD and you see that he or she is suffering and ready to leave this life, if you feel com-fortable with this, give that person permission to die. Tell them that although you'll surely miss them, you will be able to go on without them and you will be okay. People who are deathly ill often hang on and on for fear that their loved one will not be alright without them.

Treatment

Some medications that relieve pain and anxiety are also respira-tory depressants and doctors hesitate to prescribe them for people with COPD. Discuss this with your doctor and your hospice nurse, keeping in mind that *care and comfort is the goal*. The person who is dying – of any illness or disease – has the right to be as pain free and as comfortable as possible.

People with COPD are fighters. They are brave and strong, and they just don't quit. But, when the fight is gone and the strength is no longer there, they should be able to choose the path that's best for them.

Added Insight

Dale's story

This is the story of Dale who had pulmonary fibrosis, which is a chronic restrictive (not obstructive) lung disease. Even so, to anyone with a chronic, progressive, incurable disease Dale's story has not only great meaning, but a lot of heart. It is told by his wife, Mary.

First, after diagnosis, came the many questions – but wanting only the answers we wanted to hear. Then came the time frame – how long can he (we) be active, how will this progress, how will his last days be, and what kind of death can he expect? Some of these questions can be answered by qualified professionals. Others can be answered only as time progresses.

Dale often remarked what a cruel disease this was – yet our days together became very special – a new interdependence, with me the "strong" one. How I played that strong role, wanting to give Dale the peace of mind he so pursued. My tears were inward, private, or suppressed – showing only when a tender moment or happening occurred.

We learned more about oxygen tanks, ice crystals, and frozen oxygen equipment parts than we thought we ever needed to know. But we handled all these "crises" only to learn a lesson for the next time.

It was the year of our forty-fifth wedding anniversary. Our children offered to give us an open house. Thinking it might not be possible in another year, we agreed. Dale had been active singing in a barbershop chorus and quartets for over thirty years. Of course, the men in his quartet were invited and he and his group sang songs all evening, even as oxygen flowed through his trans-tracheal catheter.

Many of those songs were the "old timey" ones – some were love songs sung especially to me. This was June 8. I had no idea that his life would be over on July 18 of that year. Saturday, July 13, he still sang the barbershop tunes he so loved, even though he had to sneak extra breaths!

Whatever choices were left to us, after losing much of his mobility, we chose to do as much as possible. Not always a conscious decision, but one we had always embraced. Do it, see it, as much of life as we could encompass.

Our choice was to take a family vacation, a cruise. On June 20 Dale, our daughter Karen, and I started out on the drive from Michigan to Miami, Florida. We took with us our 100-gallon oxygen reservoir, two portable tanks, water, towels, basin (for the inevitable freeze-up of the oxygen ports), suitcases, coolers, and all the usual paraphernalia needed for a long trip. On Sunday the 23rd we boarded a ship with two couples of our three children to cruise for a week.

Much of Dale's time on the cruise was spent being chauffeured (in a wheelchair) by various family members. Each was jealous of his turn to chauffeur Dad. Sitting out on deck usually turned into naptime, but Dale always woke up in time to go to the casino and with plenty of quarters in hand, have his chair adjusted in front of a "hot" slot machine. When he would win ten dollars, he was as delighted as a little kid, even though it had cost him twenty or so to win!

After all the hard work on that trip, loading and unloading all the paraphernalia, wheeling Dale into men's bathrooms (hoping they weren't already occupied), dealing with the inconvenience of handicapped travel – it was worth it to hear Dale say, "I'm so glad we went. I had such a good time!" Reward enough! We now had memory treasures to store up for a time when only memories would be left.

After returning from our trip July 1 we saw a rapid descent in health. Dale made a call to his pulmonary rehab program and spoke with the respiratory therapist who had worked with him there for many years. After telling her about the cruise, he said, "I won't be coming back. I'm sorry. I just can't do it anymore."

She responded, "Dale, I'd like to urge you to keep on coming, but I know this has been really rough for you. And you've been the one going through it. I'm not in your shoes, so I will just say that I respect your decision – and that we will miss you."

Another ending for my dear Dale. How could we give up more? There was so little left! The anxiety attacks never seemed to leave him, and the dependence on me and others grew. Rides in his wheelchair were given even though he protested, "I don't know how long I can do this," and ended in wanting to be left out in the sun and warm breezes.

Hospice had been summoned and we faced the certainty of imminent death. How can we face a final parting? Partners for forty-five years – now partners no more – not imaginable!

Those final moments of our life together began when I called our hospice nurse to help me get Dale out of the wheelchair and back into the hospital bed. He wanted the head of the bed made level (he hadn't slept on a level surface for some time) and when he was in his bed he breathed irregularly for a few breaths, and my love, my lover, and my friend found his sought-after peace. I was able to say good-bye and assure him of my love, and he left me for a distress-free, celestial place.

Words of wisdom after my experiences with disease, dying, and death would be:

- Love each other as unconditionally as humanly possible.
- Tell each other of your love and appreciation.
- Live your lives as fully as your physical condition will allow.
- Let other loved ones support and care for you both.

Your Turn

Key points, or...if you don't remember anything else from this chapter, remember this:

- Dying is a part of life – for every one of us.
- Dying with COPD is all about doing so with personal dignity and having your wishes (not someone else's) carried out in your final days.
- Make your wishes known by telling loved ones what you want. Then put it into writing.

Ask yourself this:

- Have I given thought to my passing, and talked with my loved ones about it?
- Do I have an advance directive? For more on advance directives, see chapter October – Week 2.

This week:

Find an activity each day that gives you joy in that moment and write it down in the chart on the next page. On the seventh day look back on your list and see all those good things.

If you answered "no" to the advance directive question, start to think about this and set up a time to talk with your doctor, a close family member or friend, or both. Consider sharing your story using the suggestions above.

June – Week 3

Your Questions about Oxygen with Answers from Lung Professionals

Francis Adams, MD, Robert Sandhaus, MD, PhD, FCCP Helen Sorenson, MA, RRT, CPFT, FAARC

"Experience tells you what to do; confidence allows you to do it."

~ Stan Smith

Below are ten of the most common internet search questions on oxygen, and answers from top lung professionals. Our sincere thanks to them for making the time to answer these important questions!

Always consult with your health care provider about any changes in oxygen use. Discuss this information with your doctor so he or she can advise you appropriately for your individual situation. This is for information only and not intended as medical advice.

The first three questions were answered by Dr. Francis Adams.

1.) What is a normal blood oxygen level?

Oxygen levels are commonly measured by two techniques. The first is a blood gas in which a blood sample is taken directly from an artery. This is the most accurate assessment of oxygen. The normal oxygen level using this technique is 80-100 (mmHg).

The second technique is bloodless and is called pulse oximetry. The result here is not a direct measurement of oxygen but rather represents the percentage of hemoglobin that is saturated with oxygen. Hemoglobin is a protein in the blood that carries oxygen to the tissues. A light sensor is used which is commonly placed on a fingertip. Pulse oximetry is not as accurate as a blood gas and can be influenced by temperature and circulation. The normal oxygen saturation is 95-100%.

2.) Can I get addicted to oxygen?

I do not believe that you can become addicted to oxygen in the sense that one becomes compelled to use it as in alcoholism or heroin addiction. Many patients do become oxygen "dependent" because their bodies are unable to function without the use of oxygen supplementation. Oxygen is life sustaining and its use prolongs life and improves its quality in individuals with inadequate levels.

3.) How do I know when I need oxygen?

The most common symptom of a need for oxygen would be shortness of breath. When oxygen levels fall in the blood, nerve receptors in the neck recognize the deficiency and send distress signals to the brain. The result is the sensation of shortness of breath and an increase in the number of respirations per minute (rapid breathing). When oxygen levels are low a bluish hue might be noticed in the lips or fingertips, which is called cyanosis. Any patient experiencing shortness of breath should have an oxygen measurement.

The next three questions were answered by Dr. Robert Sandhaus.

4.) Can too much oxygen hurt me?

There are some very specific situations in which it can be harmful to take in too much oxygen. However, for most people with COPD who receive oxygen through a nasal cannula, the answer is no, too much oxygen won't hurt you. However, using too much oxygen is wasteful and can cause dryness and other discomforts.

So, what are the situations in which too much oxygen can be harmful? The brain regulates breathing based on the amount of carbon dioxide in the blood. Some individuals with very severe COPD retain carbon dioxide in their blood and the brain then begins to regulate breathing based on the amount of oxygen in the blood. Giving such a person too much oxygen can actually turn off their drive to breathe and cause life threatening respiratory arrest. Therefore, people with very severe COPD should check with their healthcare provider about whether they are at risk for this type of reaction to too much oxygen.

There are two other situations in which too much oxygen can be harmful. The first is giving high flow oxygen to newborn babies, which can cause blindness. The second is giving 100% oxygen to someone for a very long time, usually through a tube into the trachea (windpipe) attached to a breathing machine or ventilator. Receiving very high amounts of oxygen over many days in this manner can injure lung cells.

5.) Can *not enough* oxygen hurt me?

If you need supplemental oxygen, not getting enough oxygen to raise your blood levels of oxygen to an appropriate level can have very serious long-term effects. Too little oxygen causes the blood vessels in the lungs to constrict, making it more difficult for the heart to pump blood through the lungs. As a result, the pressure in the blood vessels feeding the lungs can rise, a condition known as Pulmonary Hypertension. If this goes on long enough the right side of the heart, the side that sends blood to the lungs, can fail, giving you a condition called right heart failure or Cor Pulmonale.

In addition, if you don't have sufficient oxygen delivered to the tissues of the body, they can't function as they should. The organs most affected by low oxygen, in addition to the heart, are the muscles and the brain.

6.) If I use my oxygen during the night when I sleep, can it carry over into the day?

The oxygen that gets into your blood by using supplemental oxygen leaves your system within several minutes after removing your cannula. Therefore, although the oxygen you use during the night can have many long-term beneficial effects, the oxygen itself is gone from your system fairly soon after you turn off the oxygen tank or concentrator.

Many patients only need oxygen when they sleep, and their oxygen levels are fine without supplemental oxygen during the day. But if you need oxygen both at night and during the day, using it only at night, while better than not using oxygen at all, is not sufficient to keep you well oxygenated during the day.

The last four questions were answered by respiratory therapist, Helen Sorenson.

7.) I feel like I can't breathe, but they tell me my oxygen levels are normal; and

8.) I am on oxygen, but I am not breathing any better.

These are common questions, ones we hear all the time. It might make sense that if your oxygen (O_2) levels are fine, all is right with the world, but that is not always the case.

Questions #7 and #8 are basically the same. Dyspnea, or the sensation of difficult breathing does not always correlate well with the amount of O_2 in the blood – so oxygen levels may be fine, but breathing is hard. When O_2 levels are okay and you still feel like you "can't breathe," your dyspnea is likely caused by anxiety (often a result of feeling not able to breathe). This can be a vicious cycle. This is where pursed-lips breathing is most useful, because is slows down breathing, relaxes you and often makes breathing easier. Another hint to decrease the sensation of difficult breathing is to sit in front of a fan – cool air facial stimulation decreases the sensation of dyspnea. Pulmonary rehabilitation patients tell me time and time again that the most important thing they learn from rehab is how to breathe correctly.

9.) Can oxygen in my nose get in even when I have clogged sinuses?

That depends on the degree of obstruction/sinus congestion. If the nasal passages are completely swollen/blocked, a cannula might not be as effective; but if your sinuses are congested a little, you are likely breathing more through your mouth, then the oxygen going into the nasal passages will be pulled into the lungs by the air coming in through the mouth. I have seen patients put their cannula in their mouth, but that does not usually make the delivery of oxygen to the lungs any more effective.

10.) How long can my oxygen tubing be before the oxygen reaching me becomes less effective?

The length of the oxygen tubing should not affect the liter flow of oxygen being delivered. It just may take a little longer for the oxygen to get to you initially – like when it is first turned on – but once it is flowing, it should remain constant.

Even though oxygen is a gas, we have to think of it in terms of being a liquid – if the pressure at the tank remains constant (which it does until the tank has less than 500 psi), the liter flow, 2 liters per minute (LPM), 3 LPM, etc., will remain constant. Think in terms of a garden hose – if the pressure/flow of water coming out of the faucet is constant, regardless of the length of the hose, the same amount of water will exit the other end. The only thing that may affect oxygen delivery is if there is an occlusion/obstruction in the tubing.

Your Turn

Key points, or…if you don't remember anything else from this chapter, remember this:

- We all need oxygen and have since the moment we were born.
- If tests show that you require supplemental oxygen, you should use it as prescribed.
- Using oxygen as directed will help prolong your life and take stress off your other major body systems.

Ask yourself this:

- Am I doing all I can to use my oxygen as prescribed?
- Have I checked with my oxygen provider to make sure the system I'm using is the best for me and my lifestyle?

This week:

If you don't already have a home pulse oximeter, talk with your doctor about getting one.

June – Week 4

COPD: Unseen and Misunderstood

"Sick lungs don't show."

~ John W. Walsh

"Which one of us is going to limp today?" said Mary Pierce to her husband Todd, as they got out of their car and walked towards the entrance of the store. They were used to getting dirty looks as they parked in the handicapped parking spot.

"People use to see us getting out of the car and you just knew what they were thinking. They didn't see either of us with crutches – or a wheelchair. They didn't see my lungs, how bad they were, especially when you're young, like many of the Alpha's." (Alpha-1 Antitrypsin Deficiency is a genetically inherited form of COPD that manifests in people as early as their teens and twenties. See chapter April – Week 1: Could You Have Alpha-1?)

One of the most difficult aspects of dealing with COPD is that it is rarely understood by those who are not personally affected by it. Close family members and/or spouses may eventually learn a good bit about the devastating effects of COPD, asthma, bronchiectasis, Alpha-1 Antitrypsin Deficiency, cystic fibrosis, pulmonary fibrosis, or other chronic diseases of the respiratory system. But sadly, some never do.

Having COPD can cause disabilities that, while enormously

restricting and progressively debilitating, are not obvious to casual observers, or some friends, employers, and neighbors. All around us we find people who don't understand that there are certain things we simply can no longer physically do for ourselves. Nor do they comprehend what a price we pay for having to ask for help, or how it erodes our self-esteem.

All of us wish to maintain as much of the personal pride and dignity we can. So, what can we, as patients, do to help others understand? In my experience, education about COPD is the key to improved emotional support from our friends and loved ones. We need to take it upon ourselves, as a mission, to bring every opportunity to those around us, even to the general public, to learn about COPD.

As we learn more ourselves, we should look for ways to get that vital information to spouses, relatives, even our friends and neighbors. Help them know the symptoms of this disease, the restrictions, and what it takes to fight our way to maintain stability or to improve from an exacerbation. But we must make sure we do this with a positive attitude, reminding them of what we still can do.

We need to encourage our spouses or caregivers to join us at support group meetings, where they can listen and learn from guest speakers or from the patients themselves. Siblings are also welcome at meetings, as well as our sons and daughters.

The most important thing to remember is this: We should invest our energy in positive things that we can do for ourselves, and then we'll be better able to do whatever we can to have a deeper understanding of this disease, for ourselves and others. This will go a long way toward achieving our goal of holding on to as much quality of life as possible and bringing lung disease out of the shadows.

Your Turn

Key points, or…if you don't remember anything else from this chapter, remember this:

- Most of the time, COPD cannot be seen by others, making it difficult for them to understand it.
- It is up to you to help educate those close to you about your COPD and how it limits your ability to function, but also about things you are able to do.

Ask yourself this:

Have I explained to those I care about what COPD is and how it affects me?

This week:

Invite a close friend or family member to come with you to your next support group meeting or show them a website and/or online forum for people with COPD.

Here's more help:

But You Don't Look Sick www.butyoudontlooksick.com

July – Week I

Learning to Breathe Again –
Part I: Pursed-Lips Breathing

"Learn something new each day."

~ Iris Carlyle

Always check with your doctor or respiratory healthcare professional before starting any new technique or exercise. This is for information only and not intended as medical advice.

You'd think that breathing would be as easy as inhaling and exhaling; something you wouldn't have to think about at all. But as a person with COPD, you know that at times staying in control of your breathing can be very difficult – sometimes almost impossible. This week we're going to talk about proper breathing techniques with COPD.

If you have COPD, there have been changes in your lungs and possibly, in your chest, that keep you from being able to breathe as you once did. To understand proper breathing techniques and how to use them effectively, you first need to know what's going on in your lungs.

COPD is a combination of emphysema and chronic bronchitis. Alveoli (air sacs) that are stretched out can cause stale air to get trapped in the lungs, causing them to overinflate. This is called hyperinflation. Blockages in the bronchial airways can also cause air trapping. When this happens your lungs are actually too big, they're crowded inside your chest and don't have a lot of room to move. To breathe with over-inflated lungs can take a whole lot of work with not a whole lot of results. This is one of the main reasons why breathing with COPD can be so hard.

Also, in COPD, the inside walls of your bronchial airways (the tubes inside your lungs that the air travels through) can become weak and collapse. I don't have to tell you that if your airways collapse, that's a problem that can make breathing even harder.

There are two main breathing techniques to help when you have COPD. Each of these techniques works to compensate for specific things that have gone wrong with the mechanics of breathing, brought on by COPD. One method is pursed-lips breathing (PLB) and the other is diaphragmatic breathing (DB), also called abdominal, or belly breathing. This week we're going to talk about pursed-lips breathing.

Let's review the problems and then talk about how PLB helps.

Problem:

Weak airway walls make it more likely for bronchial airways to collapse, preventing the air from getting out. When you huff and puff, you breathe out too hard and this can collapse weak airways.

Solution:

With PLB done correctly, you create "back pressure" on the inside walls of the airways, holding the airways open longer.

Problem:

Over inflation of the lungs causes air trapping. The lungs stretch out, lose their elasticity, and become crowded inside the chest.

Solution:

Using proper PLB helps you get rid of more of the stale, trapped air. Although you can't return your lungs to a normal size, by doing PLB you can help slow down the rate of developing even more air trapping.

Problem:

Carbon dioxide (CO_2), the waste product of breathing, can build up because there is too much stale air trapped in your lungs. Retaining too much CO_2 can throw off your essential acid/base balance and affect other body systems.

Solution:

Exhaling for a longer period of time with correct PLB can rid your lungs of more CO_2.

Problem:

Huffing and puffing with exertion is exhausting and frustrating and can lead to feelings of anxiety, even panic.

Solution:

Proper PLB allows a person with COPD to have greater endurance and activity tolerance, and also experience a feeling of being more calm and in control.

This information is not to be substituted for medical advice. Always consult with your doctor before starting any new technique or exercise. These breathing techniques should be demonstrated and taught by a respiratory health professional, and when beginning, should be practiced by the patient for a few minutes at a time, a few times a day. Feel free to bring this information to your doctor and ask him or her if working with these breathing retraining techniques would be appropriate for you.

What is pursed-lips breathing (PLB), and how is it done?

PLB can be the first line of defense used by people with COPD when trying to recover from, or avoid, shortness of breath. It involves breathing in through the nose and exhaling with the lips pursed, as if you are going to whistle. How hard do you blow out? It's simple. Blow out with the same force that you would use to cool hot soup on a spoon. Blow hard enough to cool it, but not hard enough to blow it off the spoon.

Here is a start on learning pursed-lips breathing

Start by relaxing your shoulders, and while still sitting up straight, let your shoulders fall as low as possible. For people with COPD, it is common to experience a lot of upper body tension. You will not be able to do breathing retraining effectively if your shoulders are high up and tense.

Pursed-lips breathing

1. Inhale slowly through your nose.
2. Purse your lips, or pucker them gently, as if you are going to whistle.
3. Breathe out slowly while keeping your lips pursed.
4. Take twice as long to breathe out as you do to breathe in. For example, if you breathe in for a count of two seconds, breathe out for a count of four seconds.
5. Never force your air out. Just let it flow out through your pursed lips.

Pursed-lips breathing will help you:

- Slow down your breathing.
- Get rid of more of the stale, trapped air, and carbon dioxide (CO_2).
- Be in control of your breathing, instead of your breathing controlling you!

If done properly, using the right breathing techniques will go a long way in helping you move more air and stay in control of your breathing.

Your Turn

Key points, or...if you don't remember anything else from this chapter, remember this:

- Pursed-lips breathing can help you control your breathing instead of letting your breathing take control over you.
- Never hold your breath!
- Keep your shoulders down and as relaxed as possible.
- Use PLB whenever you exert yourself.
- If you work on PLB regularly, it will eventually come naturally without having to think about it.

Ask yourself this:

When I'm short of breath, am I able to gain control over my breathing with PLB?

This week:

If pursed-lips breathing is new to you, or if you don't use it regularly, ask your doctor if it is alright for you to try. If so, practice it for a few minutes five to ten times each day.

Based on the article *Pursed-Lips Breathing: Pucker Up and Breathe Easier* written by Jane M. Martin, BA, LRT and published on COPDConnection.com. Copyright 2008, HealthCentral. All rights reserved. http://www.healthcentral.com/copd/c/19257/18835/lip-breathing-breathe

July – Week 2

Learning to Breathe Again – Part II: Diaphragmatic Breathing

"When somebody says to me – which they do, like, every five years – 'How does it feel to be over the hill?' my response is, 'I'm just heading up the mountain.'"

~ Joan Baez

I hope you've read the July – Week 1 chapter about pursed-lips breathing. If you haven't, please do, because although these two breathing techniques can be done independently, you'll get the most benefit if you learn them together. As always, check with your doctor or respiratory health professional before starting any new technique or exercise. This is for information only and not intended as medical advice.

If you have COPD, diaphragmatic breathing (DB) is another important breathing technique to learn. It is also called belly, or abdominal, breathing. Doing diaphragmatic breathing correctly can mean the difference between huffing and puffing, and struggling your way through each day, or being in control of your breathing as you do the things you want, and need, to do.

First, let's review why we're even talking about learning how to breathe. You might be thinking, "I've been breathing since the moment I was born so why am I suddenly supposed to 'learn' how to breathe?" The answer is simple. If you have COPD there have been changes in your lungs and possibly, in your chest, that cause you to no longer be able to breathe as you once did.

So, what's going on in your lungs? Some of this material is a review from chapter March – Week 4: A Look at the Lungs – How are they Supposed to Work and What Went Wrong? When lungs become damaged from cigarette smoking or other hazards in the environment, the elastic fibers within them start to deteriorate and the lungs begin to lose their elastic recoil – their ability to *get air out* effectively. You can think of this by comparing a balloon to a paper bag. The air in the balloon comes out easily because the balloon is elastic. A paper bag is not.

Over the years the loss of your lungs' elastic recoil gets worse and the lungs develop *air trapping and over inflation*. This means your lungs become bigger than they should be, which leads to trouble because the excess, stale air compresses functioning lung tissue so it can't do the job it should. Kind of like when the air bag in your car inflates and is pressing on your chest. When your lungs are too big for the inside of your chest, it's crowded in there and your lungs have trouble expanding and recoiling. Also, when this happens your diaphragm, which is supposed to be in the shape of a dome, becomes flatter, putting you – and your lung movement – at a mechanical disadvantage.

When the natural function of lung movement is less effective, you automatically begin to recruit the muscles around your collarbone, your neck, and between your ribs. Using these muscles to breathe not only takes a lot of energy but it can make you sore and tense in your shoulders and back. In addition to this, you're not using that most efficient muscle of breathing, the strongest breathing muscle you have, your diaphragm, to do most of the work. More work of breathing combined with less efficient lung movement adds up to a whole lot of effort and fatigue without a lot of results!

Problem:

The diaphragm becomes flattened at rest. It works best when it is in a dome shape.

Solution:

Diaphragmatic breathing can help strengthen that muscle to work more effectively even though it's at a mechanical disadvantage.

Problem:

Rapid, shallow breathing.

Solution:

Correct diaphragmatic breathing is achieved with slower, deeper breathing.

Problem:

Increased use of accessory breathing muscles.

Solution:

Better use of the diaphragm makes it less necessary to use inefficient accessory muscles.

Diaphragmatic (Belly or Abdominal) Breathing

Your diaphragm is a large, flat sheet of muscle just below your rib cage and above your abdomen, or belly. Your diaphragm was meant to do most of the work of breathing, but people with COPD struggle and tend to huff and puff, causing them to use the weaker muscles around the collarbone and between the ribs. By using your diaphragm when you breathe, you help your lungs expand more fully so they take in more air with less effort.

When the diaphragm flattens, pulling on the bottoms of your lungs, your abdomen should extend. Yes, just like your tummy is looking bigger. When you breathe out correctly, the diaphragm should go up, pushing on the bottoms of your lungs, helping you get rid of the stale, trapped air.

Always consult with your doctor before starting any new technique or exercise. These breathing techniques should be demonstrated and taught by a respiratory health professional, and when beginning, should be practiced for a just a few minutes at a time, a few times a day. Show this information to your doctor and ask him or her if doing these breathing techniques would be appropriate for you. This is for information only and not intended as medical advice.

Diaphragmatic breathing can be a hard concept to understand and a difficult technique to master. It takes practice, but it's worth it! Learning it works best in a reclining position. Here are the basic steps:

1. Relax your shoulders. Drop them down as low as they'll go.
2. Put your hands on your abdomen with your fingers overlapped, but not intertwined, just below your ribs.
3. Breathe in slowly through your nose, making your abdomen push out while you breathe in. (Remember to keep those shoulders down!)
4. Breathe out slowly, about twice as long as you breathed in, using pursed lips. Gently with your hands, push your belly in and think about blowing out all that stale air.
5. Practice this from time to time throughout the day for a few minutes at a time.

If you experience muscle soreness or fatigue with this technique it is probably because you are either working too hard at it or not doing it correctly. That's why you should learn this method only with the supervision of a person who specializes in proper breathing techniques. Once you catch on, you will breathe easier and feel less tired. Using this technique, along with pursed-lips breathing, will go a long way in helping you have less shortness of breath with exertion, and help you get through anxious episodes.

One more word of caution – be careful of breathing methods or devices you may hear about, read about in magazines, or see on the internet. Remember, if something sounds too good to be true, it probably is! Before you spend your money on any breathing aid not ordered by your doctor, ask your doctor or a respiratory health professional about it.

Using proper breathing techniques with COPD can mean the difference between struggling to get through your day – and being in control and breathing easier.

Added Insight

A tip on practicing diaphragmatic breathing from respiratory therapist Helen Sorenson

One of the "fun" things I did with my patients in support group was to have them lie down on the floor, put a box of tissues (light weight) on their belly and have them try to make it fall off just by doing their belly breathing. Strengthening the abdominal muscles is such a good exercise, as those abdominals can help out the diaphragm, which loses some of its strength as a result of the disease process. Actually, even aging alone causes us to lose strength in our diaphragm – so we (those of you over sixty like me) can all benefit from performing these exercises.

I have also seen therapists put added weight on patients' abdomens in rehab to make them work the abdominal muscles. Doing belly breathing and pursed-lips breathing at the same time has been shown to reduce dyspnea (shortness of breath), improve relaxation, and increase the efficiency of breathing. All of this can help you have more control over your breathing and eliminate some anxiety.

Your Turn

Key points, or…if you don't remember anything else from this chapter, remember this:

- Changes in your lungs lead to inefficient breathing patterns just when you have less energy and oxygen available.
- Doing diaphragmatic breathing can mean the difference between huffing and puffing or being in control of your breathing.

Ask yourself this:

What breathing muscles am I using the most to help my air go in and out?

This week:

If diaphragmatic breathing (DB) is new to you, or if you don't use it regularly, practice it for a few minutes five times each day. DB is harder to master than PLB so if you get tired or frustrated, just give yourself a break and try again later.

Based on the article *Breathe Easier with Diaphragmatic Breathing* written by Jane M. Martin, BA, LRT and published on COPDConnection. com. Copyright 2008, HealthCentral. All rights reserved. http://www. healthcentral.com/copd/c/19257/19537/breathe-diaphragmatic

July – Week 3

Relaxation

"A field that has rested gives a bountiful crop."

~ Ovid

Always consult with your doctor before starting any new technique or exercise. Show this information to your doctor and ask him or her if doing these relaxation techniques would be appropriate for you. This is for information only and not intended as medical advice.

"Relaxing" or "relaxation," mean different things to different people. For some, relaxing means coming home from work, taking their shoes off, sipping a drink, reading the newspaper, playing a game on the computer, or watching TV. While for others, relaxation is that nap they sneak in during the day. Some people find it relaxing to go for a run. For others, resting in peaceful surroundings, without anger and irritation, is relaxation. Actually, physical and mental relaxation mean undoing the physical and mental stress or tension you are experiencing at the time.

There are people apprehensive of the word relaxation, viewing it with suspicion and hesitancy. They fear that if they begin to relax, they will become lazy, unproductive, and lose the "fight" in them. Nothing could be further from the truth. Relaxation can nourish you, make you stronger and help you be better prepared to fight any challenge you might face.

We do not always recognize when we are tense, and this is especially true if you have COPD. Most people who are habitually tense have been that way for many years. Tension and stress have become the natural state of their body and mind. They are unaware of the tension they carry with them day and night, twenty-four hours a day, seven days a week. If they were asked "Are you tense?" They would say "No! I'm okay," because they have not truly experienced relaxation and thus do not know the difference.

Benefits of relaxation

I often wonder, with so many effective relaxation methods available today, why people tend to use sleeping pills and chemical relaxants. Relaxation techniques can help us to sleep and feel better, naturally. While the effect of sleeping pills and chemical relaxants wears off over time as one develops a tolerance for them, with relaxation techniques, the more you use them, the more effective they become.

When you can deepen your relaxation, you can enjoy it even more. And unlike sleeping pills or other chemical relaxants, there are no bad side effects of relaxation techniques! Regular practice of mental and physical relaxation may help you, also, to breathe more easily and relieve some of your breathing discomfort.

It takes about fifteen to twenty minutes to complete a full relaxation session. It is more effective to learn relaxation at first, by using full relaxation methods. If your stress level, pain, or another type of challenge is really high, do two or three full sessions a day. One session a day is good, two times better, and three times is excellent.

Once basic relaxation skills are acquired, you will be able to relax quickly and easily without taking so much time. Practice full and short methods frequently. Quick methods take the wind out of the sails of the stress ship. When you are in the middle of a challenging situation, you can apply quick methods right then and there, in the face of the situation.

Record and play

You may record the scripts of the relaxation sessions in your own voice and play them during your relaxation session. After sufficient practice these words will become part of you and you won't need to play them.

Full Relaxation Method (15-20 minutes)

Preparation for relaxation

Relaxation exercise can be done lying down or sitting. If you prefer to lie down, make sure you have proper pillow support under your neck and lower back or knees, if needed. Or you can sit with your arms and hands in your lap or on your thighs, with your back, neck, and head straight but relaxed. Make yourself comfortable.

Affirmation

Silently or aloud say to yourself with conviction, "I will do my best to relax physically and mentally in spite of annoying problems, such as outside noise, cough, shortness of breath, or pain. Thoughts, feelings, and sensations may interrupt me, but I can quickly bring my mind to the part of my body I want to relax. Staying relaxed and calm, I simply bring my attention to each part of my body."

Begin

- Feet relax...relaxing soles of my feet, toes and ankle joints.
- Legs from ankle joints to knee joints.
- From knee joints to thigh joints.

- Relaxing pelvis...abdomen...midsection...and chest.
- Relaxing, my hips...lower back...mid-back...and upper back.
- My whole upper body relaxes...front...back...from inside... from outside...my entire upper body relaxes.
- Aaah! (Sigh while exhaling.)
- Relaxing shoulders, shoulder pads and the shoulder blades... now the space between the shoulder blades.
- Relaxing my upper arms from shoulder joints to elbow joints.
- Upper arms and elbows, lower down towards the hips.
- Forearms to wrists.
- Hands relax all the way down to my fingertips.
- The top of my hands and palms relax.
- Nice, lazy, relaxing feeling of warmth and heaviness...from fingertips all the way up through my arms and shoulders.
- The back of my neck and head relaxes.
- All the tiny and large muscles in my neck and throat relax.
- Feeling of relaxation spreads over to the nape of my neck... the back of my head...over my entire scalp...down to my forehead.
- Forehead feels smooth like the touch of lavender or a cool breeze.
- The feeling of relaxation flows down my face.
- Nostrils relax and feel more open than before.
- Any blockages in the upper part of my nose relax and shrink.
- Sinuses relax and open up.
- My jaw relaxes.
- Gums, teeth, tongue, hard and soft palate, and my throat relax from inside.
- I observe my breathing without trying to change it in any way.

While inhaling through my nose, silently saying, "In 1-2."
While exhaling through pursed lips, silently saying, "Out 1-2-3-4."

"In 1-2…"Out 1-2-3-4."
"In 1-2…"Out 1-2-3-4."
"In 1-2…"Out 1-2-3-4."
"In 1-2…"Out 1-2-3-4."
"In 1-2…"Out 1-2-3-4."

I imagine I'm breathing in as if through the crown of my head and breathing out through the toes and the soles of my feet.

"In 1-2…"Out 1-2-3-4."
"In 1-2…"Out 1-2-3-4."
"In 1-2…"Out 1-2-3-4."
"In 1-2…"Out 1-2-3-4."
"In 1-2…"Out 1-2-3-4."

- My neck and shoulders become more relaxed and looser.
- Shoulders are back and down...shoulder blades slightly lowered towards the mid-back.
- My diaphragm is soft, relaxed and increased in length. It contracts and relaxes as I breathe.
- When I exhale, my diaphragm goes up higher than ever before and pushes up against the bottom of my lungs, expelling the air more completely.
- I picture my diaphragm attached to my lower ribs as a sheath, separating my abdomen from my lower chest.
- As my diaphragm moves, the lower ribs also move. Muscles between the ribs are becoming strong and flexible, helping my ribcage move.
- I exhale softly and slowly. My diaphragm on both sides goes up like a dome, pushing up on the bottom of my lungs.
- The center of my diaphragm goes up and massages my heart at the same time.

- As my diaphragm moves up, my lower ribs drop slightly lower, down towards my hips.
- I exhale and feel my diaphragm moving up towards the lungs.
- As I breathe in softly and gently, my diaphragm goes down... side ribs spread out and up like wings on both sides.
- My ribcage lifts, lumbar curve arches...at the same time, my abdomen between my navel and breastbone tip lengthens.

Visualization

Picture for a few minutes in your "mind's eye" any of the following: The place you would like to be right now or the time of your life you loved and enjoyed most. Spend as much time as possible. Savor that time and place in your mind.

Short Relaxation (5-10 minutes)

Preparation for relaxation

Relaxation exercise can be done lying down or sitting. If you prefer to lie down, make sure you have proper pillow support under your neck and lower back or knees, if needed. Lie if you prefer, or sit, making yourself comfortable. Sit with your arms and hands in your lap or on your thighs. Keep your back, neck, and head straight but relaxed.

Affirmation

Silently or aloud say to yourself with conviction, "I will do my best to relax physically and mentally in spite of annoying problems, such as outside noise, cough, shortness of breath, or pain. Thoughts, feelings, and sensations may interrupt me, but I can quickly bring my mind to the part of my body I want to relax. Staying relaxed and calm, I simply bring my attention to each part of my body."

- Relaxing shoulders, shoulder pads and the shoulder blades... now the space between the shoulder blades.
- Relaxing the upper arms from shoulder joints to elbow joints.
- Upper arms and elbows lower down to forearms to wrists.
- Hands relax all the way down to the fingertips.
- The top of my hands and palms relax.
- Nice, lazy, relaxing feeling of warmth and heaviness from fingertips all the way up through the arms and shoulders.
- The back of my neck and head relaxes.
- All the small and large muscles in my neck and throat relax.
- Feeling of relaxation spreads over to the nape of the neck... back of the head...over my entire scalp...down to my forehead.
- Forehead feels smooth, like the touch of lavender or a cool breeze.
- The feeling of relaxation flows down my face.
- Nostrils relax and feel more open than before.
- Any blockages in the upper part of my nose relax and shrink.
- Sinuses relax and open up.
- My jaw relaxes.

While inhaling, silently saying, "In 1-2."
While exhaling, silently saying, "Out 1-2-3-4."
"In 1-2..."Out 1-2-3-4."
"In 1-2..."Out 1-2-3-4."
"In 1-2..."Out 1-2-3-4."
"In 1-2..."Out 1-2-3-4."
"In 1-2..."Out 1-2-3-4."
"In 1-2..."Out 1-2-3-4."
"In 1-2..."Out 1-2-3-4."
"In 1-2..."Out 1-2-3-4."
"In 1-2..."Out 1-2-3-4."
"In 1-2..."Out 1-2-3-4."

Your Turn

Key points, or…if you don't remember anything else from this chapter, remember this:

- It is important for us to relax, especially with COPD.
- You are probably tense, possibly *very* tense, and don't even realize it.
- Anyone can learn relaxation techniques.
- Relaxation techniques, once learned, can help you feel better and breathe better.

Ask yourself this:

When is the last time I felt truly relaxed?

This week:

Take 15-20 minutes each day to go to a quiet place and work on the full relaxation session.

July – Week 4
Keeping a Journal

"Writing in a journal each day allows you to direct your focus to what you accomplished, what you're grateful for, and what you're committed to doing better tomorrow."

~ Hal Elrod

For a long time, I've extolled the virtues of keeping a journal, and tried to encourage people in our support group to write about their experiences with lung disease. It's mentioned frequently in my book on COPD, <u>Courage and Information for Life with Chronic Obstructive Lung Disease.</u> In fact, that's how the book began; after a while, writing in my journal started me thinking about turning it into a manuscript; the reason being to provide help to others through my own perspectives as a COPD patient.

You might think that writing is only for people who are good spellers or are especially articulate; but below is a good reason why keeping a journal is good for almost anybody…and we now know that it is especially helpful to those with a chronic disease.

Some time ago a study on journaling was done at the State University of New York at Stony Brook. A report on this study* that appeared in the Journal of the American Medical Association said, "Writing about traumatic life experiences helps patients suffering from asthma or rheumatoid arthritis improve their health."

Here's how the study was done. Researchers in Stony Brook's psychiatry department worked with a group of 112 asthma and arthritis patients. They asked half the patients to spend 20 minutes daily over three days, writing either about their most stressful life events or simply about ordinary things such as their daily schedule. They didn't ask the other half of the patients (the control group) to do anything differently.

Those with arthritis who wrote about their trauma reported a 28% reduction in disease severity within four months, while the control group showed no change. Asthmatics who wrote about their trauma showed a 19% increase in lung function against no change in the control group.

"We don't want to tell people to throw away their medicines, but what this study tells us is that we need to pay attention to psychological factors when we are talking about the treatment of chronic illness."

Overall, an analysis of the findings showed that 47% of the patients who wrote about their trauma were reported by an independent physician to be clinically improved compared to 24% of the control patients.

Please understand, this is not to say by any means, that keeping a journal should replace any of your medications or treatments. But, ask yourself this, "With this information in mind, would it harm me to spend a few minutes each day writing?"

Do yourselves a favor, my friends. Invest a couple bucks in a notebook or create a journal file in your computer, and then spend some time writing each day. The blank page will listen to what you have to say, and no one else need ever read it, unless you want them to. You can express your feelings, frustrations, your fears and triumphs at your own pace, in your own way. Keep it in a private place and allow this wonderful form of self-expression to capture the thoughts that can't easily be shared out loud. Twenty minutes of writing in a journal each day is painless, harmful to no one, and doesn't really cost anything.

When I attended the funeral service of a departed member of our Cape Cod COPD Support Group, I was particularly moved that one of his daughters read from the pages of his daily journal. She said he started writing the journal to document his struggles with COPD, and to mark the really good days so he could remember them on the bad days. I'm sure that it did not occur to this man that his words would bring comfort to his family and friends after he was gone. But they did.

Even the writing I do to produce this newsletter has helped me personally, just as writing my book was cathartic for my soul. I suspect that together, these two projects are responsible for a lot of my COPD stability over the years, and for a significant lift in my spirit and my heart. Thank you for reading. I hope my writing efforts – labors of love, really – have brought and will continue to provide an equal share of comfort and healing to you, as well.

Reference: Smyth JM, Stone AA, Hurewitz A, Kaell A. Effects of Writing About Stressful Experiences on Symptom Reduction in Patients with Asthma or Rheumatoid Arthritis. *JAMA*.1999;281(14): 1304-1309.

Added Insight

Bonnie's Story

I had never been in a hospital before except a long time ago to have two babies. But then, when I found myself as a patient in the hospital because of my breathing, I wondered, "What am I doing here all hooked up to everything imaginable going into me? I was frightened. Who wouldn't be?

I knew I had to do something to help myself feel better. I had heard that keeping a journal can help when something is bothering you. So, on the way home I thought, "Okay, let's give this a try."

I got a little book. Every day in the page on the left I recorded what medicine I took, how I felt, who came to visit me, what I did, whether I wrote checks – just little things. What did I do today? How many times did I take my inhaler? Was there something good on television? It seems so insignificant, I know. But I can look back in my journal and see what exercises I was doing, and what exercises I am actually doing now. It keeps me on track.

You'd be surprised how fast a year goes, and how interesting it is to look back and see what you were doing. I was doing tai chi, walking three times, taking a nap, and I got one of these little bicycles that you sit in the chair and pedal. I did that every day. On the page on the right, I write down good things that happen. Happy things. Things I'm thankful for.

I've been doing this, let's see…well, this is my fourth year. I would encourage everyone to make a little journal. It might seem unimportant to you, but it works for me. Try it and it might work for you too!

Your Turn

Key points, or…if you don't remember anything else from this chapter, remember this:

- If you have COPD, writing in a journal each day can help you feel better.
- Writing in a journal is an easy, inexpensive way to help you stay focused and on track with caring for your COPD.

Ask yourself this:

Am I willing to try keeping a simple journal this week?

This week:

Get a lined tablet, no smaller than 5 x 7 inches. Each day write enough to fill at least half a page. You can write about your COPD, if you're having a good day, a bad day, if you went somewhere, if you exercised, or what you ate. Just write about whatever comes to mind. Make it a habit and see how you feel at the end of the week.

July – Week 5
Medications

"Experience tells you what to do; confidence allows you to do it."

~ Stan Smith

Some time ago I was teaching a series of COPD and asthma management classes to a group of home care nurses. I was explaining how important it is for pulmonary patients to understand their inhaled medications – how each one is different from the others, how each one is supposed to work, and how they can get as much benefit as possible from them.

One nurse told a story. Visiting one day with one of her COPD patients, she saw from across the room a very large ashtray (yes, an ashtray!) filled to overflowing with a variety of inhalers. She asked the patient about the use of these inhalers, and he casually said, "Oh, when I feel tight I just take a couple puffs off this one or that one or another one until I start to feel better." Yikes! Not exactly what I'd call informed or effective use of inhaled COPD medication!

When I ask patients what their inhalers do, they almost always respond by saying, simply, "They open up my lungs." Well, yes, that's true, but, what's really important for all people with COPD to know and understand is that there are different types of medications that open the bronchial airways in different ways.

This is kind of complicated, but it is not all that hard to understand, so put your thinking caps on, and grab a pencil to jot down notes if you need to. If you own this book, don't be afraid to make marks in it, circle the names of the medications you're on and underline or highlight the categories they are in. This will help you understand what each breathing medication is supposed to do. If you're borrowing this book, it's okay to make a copy of this chapter for your personal use and take notes on your copy.

The goal of this chapter is to give you a pretty good understanding of what medication does what, and how, so you can understand your own medications and take them with maximum effectiveness.

Here we go…I'm going to start out by breaking things down into major categories and then we'll continue down the lists to learn more as we go along.

Fire prevention and calling 911

There are two different, very basic, ways that medications act to open up the bronchial airways in your lungs: Prevention (Maintenance or Controllers) and Rescue, (Rescue or Relievers). For the sake of this discussion, let's use the words Prevention and Rescue and we'll refer to the medications as either Preventers or Rescuers. An easy way to understand Prevention and Rescue in breathing medications is to look at it like we look at fire.

Prevention

As a responsible person, you do your best to prevent fires. A few ways you do this is to take good care of your home, keep the electrical wires operating safely, ensure that the stove is turned off when you're not using it, and put hot matches in a ceramic dish or in water. Doing these things help prevent a fire from starting. But if you skip any of these steps, what might happen? You could have a raging fire. And we all know that it makes a lot more sense to prevent a fire than allowing one to start!

Rescue

If and when a fire does start, however, you have (or should have) a fire extinguisher handy. And we also have the 911 system to call for help. Thank goodness! But, again, if you can prevent a fire from starting – even knowing all the while that you have help to put it out – you should do it.

You can think of medication for your lungs in much the same way. You should use the prevention medications as directed to be as effective as possible and keep your bronchial airways from swelling up, having spasms, and getting tight. If, however, you do all you can to prevent this and you still run into problems, that's the time to reach for your rescue medication.

Note: Although every effort was made for this chapter to be as complete and accurate as possible in 2020, the lists here may not necessarily be all inclusive, nor up to date, when you read them. Medications come and go, although many are in use for decades. Medication brand names are listed in this chapter so you can learn about the medications you are on. Listing the brand names in no way promotes the use of one medication and/or device over another.

Inhaled Medications

Category: Preventers

Inhaled medications that work as preventers come in three different types.

- **Corticosteroids (ICS)**
- **Long-Acting Anticholinergics, or Long-Acting Antimuscarinics (LAMA)**
- **Long-Acting Beta-2 Agonists (LABA)**

I know this is sounding kind of complicated but stay with me here.

Corticosteroids reduce inflammation, or swelling, on the insides of your bronchial airways. Think of it in this way…ten people can be in one room, breathing the same air. Each person may have a different reaction to what is in the air. Some would be fine while others might develop tight breathing because their bronchial airways are more sensitive than others.

Likewise, let's say ten people go to the beach on the same day. Each person might have a different reaction to the sun. Some might tan and some might burn. If you are the one who gets sunburn, would it make sense to go home at the end of the day and put on sunscreen? Of course not! You can think of corticosteroids as sunscreen for the insides of your sensitive bronchial airways. They are preventers. They should be taken every day to keep bronchial airways from becoming inflamed and swollen on the insides.

Inhaled Corticosteroids (ICS)

Alvesco®
Arnuity Ellipta®
Asmanex®
Flovent®
Pulmicort®
Qvar Redihaler®

Anticholinergics, or Antimuscarinics, block the message to cause spasms of the muscles in the airways of the lungs. So, they actually stop airway muscle tightening before it starts, preventing it; kind of like putting a roadblock in the way of something that could start a problem.

Long-Acting Antimuscarinics (LAMA)

Incruse Ellipta®
Lonhala Magnair®
Spiriva Handihaler®
Spiriva Respimat®
Tudorza Pressair®

Long-Acting Beta 2 Agonists relax the muscles around your bronchial airways to keep them from squeezing. Medications that are in this long-acting category do not begin to work as soon as you take them. It takes about 20 minutes before they become effective. But they should last for about twelve hours. Therefore, if you take them twelve hours apart, you should have around-the-clock coverage for preventing those muscles from acting up and squeezing your airways.

Long-Acting Beta 2 Agonists (LABA)

Brovana®
Perforomist®
Serevent®
Striverdi Respimat®

Category: Rescuers

Short (fast) -Acting Beta-2 Agonists

These medications also work to relax the muscles around your bronchial airways to keep them from squeezing. They go to work soon after you take them. This is good, but they last for only about four to six hours (with the exception of Xopenex which works for twelve hours). Remember, our goal is to use these rescue medications as little as possible. This is because it's better to keep your airways open without giving them the chance to tighten.

Short (fast) -Acting Beta 2 Agonists (SABA)

Albuterol
Proair®
Proventil®
Ventolin®
Xopenex®

Antimuscarinics block the message to cause spasms of the muscles in the airways of the lungs. So, they actually stop airway muscle tightening before it starts, preventing it; kind of like putting a roadblock in the way of something that could start a problem.

Short-Acting Antimuscarinics (SAMA)

Atrovent®
Ipratropium Bromide

Combination Inhaled Medications

Some medications are combined into one inhaler.

Combination Corticosteroids and Long-Acting Beta 2 Agonists (ICS/LABA)

Advair®
Advair Diskus®
AirDuo RespiClick®

Breo Ellipta®
Dulera®
Symbicort®
Wixela®

Combination Short-Acting Antimuscarinics and Beta 2 Agonists (SAMA/SABA)

Combivent Respimat®
Duoneb (nebulizer)®
Ipratropium Bromide/Albuterol

Combination Long-Acting Antimuscarinics and Long-Action Beta 2 Agonists (LAMA/LABA)

Anoro Ellipta®
Bevespi Aerosphere®
Stiolto Respimat®

Combination Inhaled Corticosteroid, Long-Acting Antimuscarinic, and Long-Acting Beta 2 Agonist (ICS/LAMA/LABA)

Trelegy Ellipta®

Oral Medications (tablets or capsules you swallow)

These medications are not breathed in. They are in the form of a pill you swallow. They must first go through your digestive system. Along the way, they can cause some side effects, more so than the inhaled medications that go straight to your lungs. However, oral medications still have their place in helping you breathe.

Corticosteroids are often used if you have a bad breathing episode. They work very well within a day or two and are then tapered down once the exacerbation has passed. Long-term use of oral corticosteroids should be avoided if possible. But if you have severe COPD, are on maximum use of inhalers and still having trouble getting through your day, ask your doctor about a daily low dose.

Oral Corticosteroids

Prednisone
Methylprednisolone
Medrol®
Prednisolone
Prelone®

Methylxanthines have been around for a long time and were some of the first effective breathing medications. They work well for some people but are not prescribed as often as some other medications.

Methylxanthines

Theophylline
Theo-24®
Uniphyl®

Mucolytics are medications that thin mucus, making it less thick and sticky and easier to cough up.

Phosphodiesterase 4 (PDE4) Inhibitor is a newer medication designed to decrease the number of COPD exacerbations in adults with severe COPD.
Daliresp®

Getting your breathing medications into your lungs

Different devices

There are many different inhalers, some with different types of devices. Each one calls for a specific way of activating the medication dose and breathing it in. Some inhaler devices require users to go through a number of steps before the medication is ready to be inhaled. When you get an inhaler that is new to you, ask a pharmacist or respiratory care professional who specializes in COPD to show you how to use it. Then show that person how you would use it. Ask if you are doing it right, and if you can do it better.

Different forms of medication

Medication comes out of inhalers in three different forms.
Metered-Dose Inhalers (MDIs) – Medication comes out in the form of a fine mist. The mist comes out fast, so it helps to use a spacer or holding chamber. Breathe it in with a slow, deep breath.

Soft Mist™ Inhalers (SMIs) – Medication comes out in a soft mist, more slowly than from an MDI. A spacer or holding chamber is not used with a soft mist inhaler.

Dry-Powder Inhalers (DPIs) -- Medication is in the form of a very fine powder. With the DPI the user provides the force to get the medicine out of the device and into the lungs by taking a fast, deep breath through the mouthpiece. A spacer or holding chamber is not used with a DPI.

Spacers and holding chambers

Ask a pharmacist or respiratory care professional who specializes in COPD if you should be using a spacer or holding chamber to help you breathe as much medication as possible deep into your lungs.

Avoiding side effects

Ask a pharmacist or respiratory care professional who specializes in COPD what special precautions you should take to prevent unwanted side effects such as mouth infections or raspy throat.

Timing

If your inhaled medications are in different types, it is alright to take them one right after the other. But don't take two medications that are the same type one right after the other (Ventolin and Combivent are an example of this because they both contain a Short (fast) -Acting Beta-2 Agonist. With that said, professional opinions differ on which medication to take first. Check with your doctor about when to take each of your inhaled medications for maximum benefit in your individual situation.

That's a lot to learn, but you got through it! Remember what we said about fire? Do all you can to prevent one, and hopefully you won't have to do a whole lot of rescuing. It's important for you, a person with COPD, to know and understand how your breathing medications work. Once you do, you'll have another tool to help control your breathing – and your life!

Added Insight

Melissa's story

Melissa has asthma, but many of the lessons she learned can be helpful in medication issues with COPD. Here, she tells her story.

In my freshman year of college, I had difficulty breathing while playing tennis. I just brushed it off as being out of shape. But the problems persisted to the point where I had to stop in the middle of competition because I could not breathe well. How could this be happening to me? I was overwhelmed by thoughts and fears of not being able to exercise or to play tennis in college or *ever* being able to play again.

The idea of having asthma was so very foreign to me; initially I struggled to understand how to use all the new medications I was prescribed. Embarrassed about having to use my inhalers when I played, I felt like I was showing my opponent a weakness. I tried to be very discrete so no one would know I needed an inhaler.

Once I had accepted my diagnosis, it was a challenge for me to learn how to live with asthma, but I slowly became more sensitive to understanding my body and my medications. I was put on several inhalers: one to prevent inflammation and another to stop breathing problems when they occurred.

The regimen I established worked very well for me until the fall of my junior year when my health started to steadily deteriorate. I was having difficulty breathing and, even functioning for that matter. Nothing was making me feel better. In fact, I was getting worse. It got to the point where I could not function at the normal daily level. While experiencing a lot of fatigue and chest pain, I had difficulty breathing, preventing me from attending classes, playing tennis, and going about everyday life activities.

My lowest of lows came one day while on the tennis court. I had to default a match because an asthma attack occurred on the court. This was devastating for me; it happened in front of all my teammates who were equally as scared and concerned as I was. Forced to quit, I felt like I had lost control over the functioning of my body. *I had hit my rock bottom point and right then and there I decided I was going to beat this thing before it beat me. I was going to take control again of my body and my life!*

Finally, I was referred to a pulmonologist and started on a myriad of new medications. It was he, the lung specialist, who taught me how to use a peak flow meter and to record my daily progress on peak flow charts. Even though this was all foreign to me, I now had the tools I needed to succeed. All I had to do was follow through. I realized that carrying out his instructions was necessary for me to make progress, and at that point, I was willing to do *anything* to get better.

I became a lot less shy about people around me knowing I had asthma, for both their sake and mine; and, in fact, it soon became my desire to educate them. So, I explained to my college housemates and teammates what asthma was, what it was doing to my body and how they should react if an emergency situation arose.

Managing my asthma was also an education process for me to learn about myself, to learn about my triggers, to know about my body and how it reacts, knowing when to increase or decrease my medications, and how to take proactive steps to prevent asthma episodes. I read everything I could get my hands on so I could better understand what was going on in my body.

I went back to my pulmonologist after a month of this treatment and brought my peak flow charts. I had diligently completed all sides and columns daily, just as he asked. The charts showed my roller coaster start. I experienced many ups and downs. It has been far from easy, but with my commitment and dedication to follow the regimen, it has been well worth the effort. By bringing my charts with me, the doctor could better treat me because he could see my daily progress. This said a lot more to him than, "Oh yeah, I'm doing better."

I am happy to say that my breathing is now under control. I went from defaulting matches in February of my junior year in college, to enjoying one of my most successful tennis seasons ever! I still remember the day when I thought all my athletic dreams had been lost, but I remind myself that it was possible to do what I first thought impossible.

Through this I began to appreciate things I had taken for granted.

Breathing and exercise became a privilege. I learned that just because you are given a medication, it will not fully help you unless you are determined to take it and not stop taking it, even if you feel better. Instead of putting out fires, you do your best to make sure that one never starts. If you have asthma or COPD, view your doctor as a teammate. He or she will help you if you provide the information needed.

Your Turn

Key points, or…if you don't remember anything else from this chapter, remember this:

- It is your job to understand not only what each breathing medication is supposed to do, but how it is supposed to do it. You're smart enough to understand this!
- Take your preventer medicines as prescribed, every day, even when you're breathing well. They will help keep your breathing stable.
- Have a respiratory care professional watch the way you take your inhaled medications. If you can do better, they can give you suggestions about how to get as much benefit as possible from your inhaled medications.

Ask yourself this:

- Do I know how my different breathing medications work?
- Am I using the best possible technique?

This week:

Make sure you're taking your preventer medications exactly as prescribed. If you have questions, ask your doctor or respiratory health professional. See the resource below.

Here's more help:

The COPD Foundation Pocket Consultant Guide Patient Track app. www.copdfoundation.org/Learn-More/The-COPD-Pocket-Consultant-Guide/Patient-Caregiver-Track.aspx

August – Week I
Hope

It has never been, and never will be, easy work! But the road that is built in hope is more pleasant to the traveler than the road built in despair, even though they both lead to the same destination."

~ Marie Zimmer Bradley

Getting a diagnosis of COPD can be devastating. As patients, we learn that we have a progressive, incurable disease, one that no doubt will alter our life by limiting our physical abilities with shortness of breath and fatigue.

We may hear all or none of this information at the point of diagnosis. Some of us are just left to fend for ourselves. Most doctors, even pulmonologists, do not have the time or inclination to educate patients. So, we are left with huge holes in knowledge about COPD and how to manage it. And you must know, *COPD can be treated and managed*!

But by far, the worst thing left out of diagnosis is *hope*. We are rarely advised that we have a right to have hope with COPD. Even if a doctor suspects that his or her patient may have a poor prognosis, that person is still entitled to hope – that should never be taken away. In my case, I was diagnosed with COPD and told that I had between two and five years of life left. That was fourteen years ago! Even though I was prescribed supplemental oxygen 24/7 for the rest of my life (which I've faithfully used all these years), I'm still around... still kicking, still working every day, still very much alive... and glad of it!

Everyone deserves hope! But I had to find my own. I've done some of this by my involvement as an advocate for COPD'ers. Part of my own hope came from my quest for information about this disease. Part of it I found by writing my book about living with COPD. Part of it I stumbled upon by seeing others who were worse off than me. And part of it I gained by having faith in my own ability to overcome obstacles, even those caused by chronic illness. I continue to learn about COPD almost every day and I'm determined not to give in to it.

The big questions about hope usually comes a while after the initial diagnosis, after the shock of being told we have a progressive, incurable disease that's not going to go away. Shock tongue-ties us and prevents our brains from allowing us to reach out for vital information. Then, after the shock wears off a bit, we find ourselves in need of an understanding of what we, and our families, are facing.

Physicians are the ones we turn to most often when we are seized by fear of the unknown. I would like to see all pulmonary physicians add a few more basic facts to their ten-minute visit – to add words of hope by making sure that we, as patients, are aware that our life is not over just because we have COPD. We need to be encouraged to become active in the management of our disease and partners with our doctors, knowing that the goal is now stability of our disease and living as healthy and happy – and hopeful – as possible.

There are many things we can do to keep from getting worse, to prevent us from spiraling downward. We have a lung disease that is chronic and progressive, but we can choose to live our lives in ways that help us remain stable. By following our doctor's treatment program: eating a healthy diet, keeping up with an exercise routine, getting enough sleep, maintaining a social life, avoiding exposure to viruses and other harmful bugs, and keeping a positive outlook, we are on our way to stability!

When we're beginning to feel helpless, we must fight our way back to better control of our lives. How? By finding different ways to accomplish our goals, even if we are limited in our physical strength. We might not be able to do what we once did, in the same way we did it, but that doesn't mean we can't do lots of things.

No one should be without hope, ever! It's a ladder to hold onto. It is a reason to get up in the mornings. It gives us reason to smile. It lets us reach out to help others. It helps us sleep at night. Having hope gives us insight into what is most important in our lives. But most of all, hope provides us with inspiration, encouragement, and strength to face each day.

Added Insight

Steve's thoughts on hope.

Growing up just outside Chicago, Steve Reitveld's life was going along just as planned. He had graduated from high school, had a lot of friends, was involved in activities at church, and had just gone to baseball try-out camp. As an only son, he was poised to carry on the successful family business. But in a moment, his life changed. He was injured while working with his father on the family farm and the result of his injury was that, at age 20, Steve became a quadriplegic. Although Steve doesn't have pulmonary disease per se, he has experienced numerous health challenges over the years, including a pacemaker, colostomy, and tracheotomy with oxygen, as well as several bouts of pneumonia and a collapsed lung. Nebulizer treatments and suctioning are a routine part of his day. Here, Steve's thoughts on hope.

As a person with a chronic lung disease, you might think that my injury, leaving me paralyzed, is a very bad thing and worse than what you have, but you cannot look at it that way. Sure, this is a devastating injury, but the main thing is that I still have my mind and *I'm still me*. My body is not disfigured – it still looks the same. It just cannot move. Of course, it could be worse: I could be unable to move my arms like I can now, or my mind could be damaged, but none of those things have happened, so I'm very fortunate.

I have discovered the world of computers, that they are a godsend – and my link to the outside world. Had I not been injured would I have been this involved with computers? Probably not. If I can inspire or help just one person, with words, comfort, or visiting my website, that's good. Anything I have to share or help people with, I'm happy to give. So, out of a tragedy there have been positives. Don't look at me as a person that has lost so much – but someone who has gained so much more.

And now, regarding the subject of hope. Hope is something that's hard to keep hold of, to keep in your sights when something happens to you – chronic or terminal disease, an accident – anything. At first when something devastating happens, you think there is no hope and never will be. Honestly, I did not even want to hope for anything when I was first injured. My first thoughts were to pretty much give up because, what was the point? My life was over. My plans were over. My dreams were gone. What good would, or could I be ever again?

With an injury like mine, or a chronic/terminal illness, acceptance of the situation is a key before you can begin to hope. Sure, I hope there will be a cure for paralysis – and I'm sure someday there will be – but not in my lifetime. But that doesn't mean I can't hope for something. When news comes out about new research or new discoveries, it's easy to think it will be available the next day. In truth, it could still be years away and so I have to hope – in perspective. I'm thankful for even small advances that help me deal with day-to-day living, even if it is not a cure. I can even be hopeful for something as simple as having a good day.

We've always got to have hope... have to keep that flame burning.

A lot of days this is easier said than done. The sun will keep on rising every day and we never know what that day will bring. But we have to hope that it will be good. This is why I will never give up or lose hope because I want to be around to experience everything I can.

Whether you are spiritual or not, hope can still be there. On the coldest, darkest days of winter we still hope for spring. Finally, it comes. You know how you feel when you see that first flower pushing up through the snow? Without hope we have nothing. If life is a game of cards. I have been dealt this hand. It's not the hand wanted, but I will play it, I will make the best of it, and I'll never lose hope.

Steve passed away at the age of 51 from complications due to pneumonia. This essay was read at his memorial service.

Your Turn

Key points, or...if you don't remember anything else from this chapter, remember this:

- Along with getting a COPD diagnosis, you and your doctor should talk about what you can hope for.
- It is good, and it is right, to have hope – for something – no matter how small, or no matter how bad things are.

Ask yourself this:

What can I hope for? Is there something coming up that I can look forward to?

This week:

Start each day with one new hope for that day, no matter how small.

August – Week 2

Worry

"Worry is interest paid on trouble before it comes due."

~ William Ralph Inge

The origin of the word "worry" offers interesting insights regarding the nature and function of worry. The English words, "worrowen," "wirien," and "Wyrgan," mean "to choke" or "to strangle." In Medieval English the verb "worry" also meant "to gnaw," or to continually bite or tear something. Worries and chronic anxiety gnaw at us and, bit by bit, wear away our inner security and peace of mind.

You may be a person with COPD who had an anxiety disorder prior to developing COPD or developed one after the onset of the lung impairment. You may have had a Generalized Anxiety Disorder (GAD) from very early on, long before you developed COPD.

You may have been born with what is called "anxious temperament." According to temperament-related research, perhaps 20% of children are born with anxious temperament. Out of the 20% anxious temperament children, some will develop one or more anxiety spectrum disorders, notably GAD, phobias, panic attacks or Obsessive Compulsive Disorder. If you have excessive anxiety or concern associated with breathing difficulty, you should get an evaluation for a possible underlying disorder.

In some cases, worrying is a symptom of an anxiety disorder, depressive disorder, or a result of a deeply painful life event, such as betrayal of trust, abandonment, severe humiliation, or abuse.

If you're a worrier, you should know that to a great extent, you have a choice regarding what you think. You have the power to fight off negative and disturbing thoughts that invade your mind. You can do this by learning what you're dealing with, facing the worry monster, and breaking the hold it has on you.

Worrying is to chew over and over again that which has already been chewed. Worrying has a repetitive and obsessive quality about it. A worrier is obsessed with negative outcomes and pitfalls. A worrier imagines every misfortune that might come along. Oh, those errors, accidents, and all possible bad things that can go wrong! Remember, some of our demons are of our own making.

Do you have a worry problem?

- Have you begun to worry more than you ever did?
- Do you worry more than others do?
- Do you tend to multiply the possibilities of what can go wrong?
- On an average day, over the past month, what percentage of the day did you feel worried?
- Have you frequently been so worried that you kept on tossing and turning in bed and couldn't sleep?
- Have you ever been told, "Stop worrying! Relax!"

If you answered "yes" to any of these questions, don't worry, we will provide tips to help you cut down on your worry time. Read on!

I am sure that after worrying all night long you find yourself in the morning exactly in the same situation you were in the night before, except more sleepy and tired! In spite of worrying all night, you didn't solve anything, learn anything new, or acquire anything new, except perhaps a headache. God gave us the ability to worry to help us assess the risks facing us, and to plan appropriate steps to meet our needs. The purpose of the "work of worrying" is summarized in the saying, "forewarned is forearmed!" But if you worry only, and don't take the required action, you never get out of the swirling waters onto the shore.

The One-Minute Manager – Tips for cutting down on the habit of worrying

If you are a chronic worrier, it means that through the practice of many years of worrying, you have become really good at it. The mind learns to have "worry spasms," or a kind of "brain hiccups" that just refuse to quit. The first few seconds you start worrying are critical to stop the ever-growing worry web. When the first worry thought strikes you, you have just a few seconds, a maximum of one minute, to break the chain of worry thoughts before your entire mind gets involved in it. Once you get too involved with your worrying thoughts, you end up in the "worry grip!" Once you're there, you might not be able to relax for the next several hours – or even the whole night.

It helps to think of worry as if those thoughts are weeds in the spring. Before you know it weeds can take over the whole garden, but you can get rid of them if you apply weed killer or pull them out of the ground as soon as you see them sprout. You can break a single stick with ease; it's difficult to break a bunch of them together.

When your mind gets involved with the action of worrying, the body gets involved, as well. Your muscles tense up and the level of stress hormones keeps rising, which fuels worrying thoughts non-stop. You can train yourself to stop worrying. Just as you train your muscles to learn a golf swing, train your brain to take a swing at the worry monster.

Here are some tips to stop the worry thoughts:

1. As soon as you catch the first worry thought, challenge it! Say something positive to yourself right away. Offer counter evidence to oppose the main thrust of your worry thoughts. Offer yourself thoughts that negate your worst fears.
2. Imagine all possible outcomes instead of the negative ones. Challenge "What if...?" thoughts with "So what..." thoughts. Also challenge your negative thoughts with a skeptical attitude and ask, "How so?"

Here is an example:

Worry thought: What if they don't come to see me anymore?
Counter thought: So, what if they don't come to see me anymore. I can do without them.

Worry thought: They may all be tired of me.
Counter thought: How so? I feel they genuinely care about me. Turn the tables on your worry thoughts!

3. If you've tried everything else and you still can't shake off your worry thoughts, get out of bed and write them down. After you write them down, read them to yourself. You may often find that your imagination is somewhat exaggerated.
4. When a worry strikes you, do something physical for five minutes such as stretch, hum, or whistle. Then sit down and write out what you were worried about; describe the actions you can take to address that problem. Note the earliest time when you can act on them.
5. Think of a positive self-affirming thought, for example, "I am a doer, not a worrier!"
6. Blow your breath into your palms and say to yourself, "I just

blew off my worry," and go to bed. The next morning, follow the actions you wrote down.

If you don't strike quickly at them, worries multiply adding to an ever-growing list of things to worry about. We worry about everything, ranging from events less likely to happen to those that are most unlikely to happen. All things are not lions and tigers, but they may *appear* so to us. Soon, the world seems to be a dangerous place. Previously, one sensed danger from just a few sources, now he or she sees it everywhere. There is no shortcut and no easy way out. The dragons need to be slain, one by one.

Chronic and excessive worrying can isolate you from others, stripping you of your social support system. Don't get so involved in the act of worrying that you can't find time to connect with others. Don't let worry isolate you from people who love you!

You can learn to extricate your life from the clutches of anxiety. You probably underestimate your own power and overestimate the danger of things that confront you. If you need to, see a therapist. If there is a traumatic event in your past that keeps gnawing at you, work through it with a counselor. Often the way to overcome pain is through it and not around it.

Give yourself a gift: Learn ways to calm your fears. As you involve yourself in new situations and new activities, preoccupation with anxiety will decrease. As you develop greater self-confidence and find your life more satisfying, you may not even need anxiety pills or worry about whether a pill is habit forming.

Knowing you have the power to choose your thoughts is one of the best kept secrets! You do have a choice regarding what you think and how you feel. Just because you have always thought and felt a certain way, doesn't mean you can't train yourself to think differently. You may not have power over the outside world, but you have the choice to decide what thoughts you think – and the power to beat the worry monster.

Your Turn

Key points, or…if you don't remember anything else from this chapter, remember this:

- If you are a chronic worrier, with or without COPD, you can learn to control your worry.
- You can choose your thoughts.
- Worry can affect your physical as well as your emotional health and wellbeing.
- It is important to stop the worry soon after it starts.

Ask yourself this:

Do I have a worry problem?

This week:

- Write down your three major worries.
- Write down your "worry thoughts" related to each of the three major worries.
- Write Down Your "counter thoughts" for each of the three major "worry thoughts."

August – Week 3

Stages of COPD: Where Am I and What Does it Mean?

"Life's trials will test you, and shape you, but don't let them change who you are."

~ Aaron Lauritsen

"You have end stage COPD," is possibly one of the most frightening – and confusing – things a person can hear. First and foremost, it's important to know that "end stage COPD" is not an official medical term. It is a label tagged onto a range of lung function numbers, a label that is becoming less and less used as time goes by.

It's only fair to tell you right now, that in this chapter you will not find a chart on the stages of COPD with corresponding FEV_1 percentages. There are resources in the "Your Turn/Here's more help" on where you can find that. You will find, though, a brief timeline on the stages of COPD. You'll learn about factors that are now playing a bigger role in determining the best course of treatment for your particular COPD. You will see an example of how three people with the same FEV_1 can have significantly different experiences over the course of their disease.

Let's take a look at a timeline on the stages of COPD to learn where those numbers come from and what are they based on.

In the late 1990s COPD was considered a major public health

problem. It was the fourth leading cause of chronic morbidity and mortality in the United States and was projected to rank fifth in 2020, worldwide. Because of this, a committed group of experts encouraged the U.S. National Heart, Lung, and Blood Institute (NHLBI) and the World Health Organization (WHO) to create and develop the *Global Initiative for Chronic Obstructive Lung Disease*, better known as GOLD.

In 2001 GOLD released the classification of COPD by stage. The basic idea was to provide doctors with, not necessarily a clinical guideline, but a strategy for the diagnosis and management of COPD. The 2001 classification of COPD severity was based on spirometry alone – the ratio of FEV_1 to FVC and the FEV_1. The FEV_1 is the Forced Expiratory Volume in the first second (the amount of air you blow out in the very *first second* in that long, forced exhalation when you take a spirometry test). The FVC is the Forced Vital Capacity (the *total* amount of air you blow out in that long breath out when you take a spirometry test). So, the classification was based on the ratio of FEV_1 to FVC and the FEV_1 matched with therapy and management for patients with stable COPD. The stages were: Stage 0: At Risk, Stage I: Mild COPD, Stage II: Moderate COPD, (there were two levels within this stage), and Stage III: Severe COPD.

Over time, the strategy was modified to a classification still known worldwide and used by thousands of healthcare providers to manage their patients' COPD on a daily basis. Stage I: Mild COPD, Stage II: Moderate COPD, Stage III: Severe COPD, and Stage IV: Very Severe COPD.

In 2011 GOLD determined that the aims of COPD treatment should be focused also on two *patient-reported outcomes*: symptoms and exacerbations (flare-ups). This was a more a multi-dimensional and patient-centered approach in addition to measuring spirometry numbers. In 2017 GOLD said that a patient's history of exacerbations seemed to play a bigger role than FEV_1 when it came to a patient's risk of future exacerbations. Spirometry was still considered very important, not only for diagnosis but also for follow-up.

Source: Global Initiative for Chronic Obstructive Lung Disease, GOLD. www.gold-copd.org.

Somewhere along the way, the "very severe" stage was labeled by some as "end stage."

That's a bit of the history of how COPD stages were first developed and how they've evolved over time. Now, we come back to one of the questions most commonly asked by people with COPD, "What stage am I in now, and what can I expect?" That's a fair question, but instead of looking on a chart and finding where your FEV_1 number puts you, its important to talk about why there's a lot more to your COPD story than that number. While you should have a spirometry test and know your FEV_1, that doesn't tell us everything. Your lung function numbers alone are not a good predictor of your symptoms or what will happen with your COPD over time.

We know now, also, that there are different types of COPD. Each type may affect how well different treatments work and how your symptoms, such as shortness of breath, may progress. If you have another condition, such as heart disease, diabetes, depression, or anxiety, this can also affect your COPD treatment and symptoms.

COPD and lung function numbers are not "one-size-fits-all"

Let's say there are three people, Tom, Jill, and Sam. They all have COPD with a FEV_1 of 35% of what is predicted for their age, height, sex, and ethnicity. You might think they all have similar symptoms or are impacted by COPD in the same way. But actually, their ability to do physical activities, their tendency to have COPD exacerbations, and even the level of oxygen in their blood are very different.

Tom can walk a longer distance than Jill, but his oxygen saturation numbers (O_2 sats) get low when he walks so he uses supplemental oxygen. Every time Sam gets a cold, it becomes a COPD exacerbation and he's pretty sick for a week. But when he's not down with an exacerbation, he can walk farther than Jill. Jill hasn't had an exacerbation for a few years and her O_2 sats are good, but she has trouble walking only a short city block. Jill and Sam both have good oxygen sats but Sam can walk farther than both Tom and Jill. How can that be? Simply put, this complex disease affects Tom, Jill, and Sam differently, although they all have COPD with the same FEV_1.

Again, we now know there are several factors that help determine the impact of COPD. Your answers to the following questions can be useful in addition to your spirometry numbers.

- If you have shortness of breath, is it at rest or only with exertion?
- Do you have a cough? If so, do you cough up mucus on most days for at least three months in a period of at least two years?
- Do you have a lower oxygen level at rest, only with exertion, or when you sleep?
- Are your lungs stretched out and larger than normal?
- Do you have any chronic conditions in addition to COPD, such as heart disease, diabetes, anxiety, or depression?
- Have you had two or more exacerbations in the past year?

Spirometry Grades

In 2014 the COPD Foundation developed a guide for the diagnosis, treatment, and management of COPD. This guide, which was not meant to be in competition with GOLD, includes Spirometry Grades (SG), also based on the ratio of FEV_1 to FVC and FEV_1. They are: SG 0: Normal, SG 1: Mild, SG 2: Moderate, SG 3: Severe, and SG U: Undefined.

In this guide, the spirometry grades, along with your history of exacerbations, breathlessness score, asthma COPD overlap (ACO), and other factors, help you and your healthcare provider consider different types of treatment. Remember, all decisions must be based on your situation, your symptoms, and the total picture of you.

Source: COPD Foundation. www.copdfoundation.org.

To summarize, if you learn that your lung function numbers are in the "very severe" range and you are told you have "end-stage COPD," it is not a death sentence! Yes, COPD is progressive and currently incurable. But your lung function numbers do not determine how long you're going to live. And they certainly don't determine how you function! If you keep up with effective management of your COPD, you can live a long time and enjoy life, even with advanced disease.

Your Turn

Key points, or…if you don't remember anything else from this chapter, remember this:

- Being told that you have "end stage" COPD is not a death sentence!
- People with the same pulmonary function numbers are not necessarily in the same condition. The way COPD impacts them may differ significantly.
- You can live a long time with advanced COPD, if you learn how to manage it effectively.

Ask yourself this:

Have you had a spirometry test done within the past two to three years, and if so, do you know your FEV_1 number?

This week:

Make a note to ask your healthcare provider if all aspects of your COPD are being considered when prescribing treatment.

Here's more help: For more information on the stages of COPD, visit: www.goldcopd.org and www.copdfoundation.org/Learn-More/I-am-a-Person-with-COPD/Stages-of-COPD.aspx.

August – Week 4

Making the Most of Living with Advanced COPD

"There are many wonderful things that will never be done if you do not do them."

~ Charles D. Gil

When you have very severe or advanced COPD, of course it's important to do your best to stay physically healthy. But we should never underestimate the value of emotional health. Below is some wisdom on how to live a full and happy life from those who know – people with advanced COPD. All these suggestions might not work for you, but if you try just one or two you might be surprised how much better you'll feel.

Get out there

It might take some effort, but make plans to go out regularly, to dinner, to your grandchild's sports event or school program, or even for a ride in the car. Feeling self-conscious about wearing your oxygen? Would you expect someone who needs glasses to drive without them? Of course not! If your doctor says you need supplemental oxygen, wear it. You'll breathe easier and put a lot less stress on your major body systems. If somebody has a problem with you wearing oxygen, that's their problem – not yours.

Don't sweat the small stuff

It may be a cliché, but really…when something starts to bug you, ask yourself, "Does it really matter all that much? Is it that much of a biggie, or can I just let it go?" Being anxious can lead to even worse shortness of breath. The simple serenity prayer offers great advice. *God grant me the serenity to accept the things I cannot change; courage to change the things I can; and wisdom to know the difference.*

Laugh

Make smiles and laughter – and sharing them – a priority. One of my most favorite things about working with people with COPD is the fun we have together, telling jokes, laughing, and kidding around. Truly, some of the best times I've ever experienced are when I'm in a room full of people with "end stage" COPD.

Record your history

Everybody has a story to tell, and we should all pass ours along, whatever our age – or our health status. Make plans with a friend or family member (maybe a grandchild) to listen as you tell your story while they record it on audio, video, or digitally. Just sit down and start talking. You'll be so glad you did!

Help others

When I was writing my first book on stories of people with COPD and other chronic lung diseases, I asked people with COPD this question: "If you could say one thing to somebody with COPD who is about to give up, what would you say?" One response was, "Do something to help someone." Wow. There are many things you still can do. Make a phone call or send a cheerful note to someone who's feeling down. Volunteer for your local hospital or public library by doing a sit-down job. Listen to a child read. Give somebody a ride to the grocery store or the doctor's office. Even if you're short of breath you can help yourself... by helping others.

Go with the flow

For people with COPD probably one of the biggest – and the most confusing – concerns is the mystery of good days and bad days. Yes, it's important to pay attention to changes in your breathing, but don't spend too much emotional energy trying to figure out why yesterday was so good and today is not. Many times, there is just no explanation. Accept that bad days are a fact of life and know that tomorrow will probably be better. One way to make the most of bad breathing days is to have a "bad-air day" box or basket stocked with quiet activities you don't always have time for – a book or magazine to read, word puzzles, jigsaw puzzles, a movie you've been meaning to watch, or a small sewing or sit-down repair project (See chapter February – Week 3: Good Days, Bad Days).

Go on vacation

Are you kidding? No, I'm not. Sure, traveling with any chronic disease takes planning, but if possible, take that trip! You'll be getting out, seeing something new, having fun, and making memories to keep.

For many people with severe COPD, moving around is a big effort. In a swimming pool you'll have the freedom to move around smoothly and easily. And yes, you can swim while wearing oxygen! If you have trouble walking a distance, rent a wheelchair or a scooter. The idea is to enjoy your getaway and see some sites – not to struggle with your breathing. (See chapter March – Week 3 for travel tips.)

Sea Puffers Cruises for people with chronic lung disease offers the support you need to travel with oxygen. 1-866-673-3019 http://www.seapuffers.com/

Don't give up – and don't forget to live!

When you have severe or very severe COPD…whatever you call it…sure, there are things you can no longer do the way you once did, *but there are many things you can do.* Whatever you do, don't forget to live! You can do it. You can live long – and well – with advanced COPD.

Based on the article, *Living Well with End Stage COPD – At Home and Away* written by Jane M. Martin, BA, LRT and published on COPDConnection.com. Copyright 2009 HealthCentral. All rights reserved. http://www.healthcentral.com/copd/c/19257/85354/living-end-stage-home

Your Turn

Key points, or…if you don't remember anything else from this chapter, remember this:

- If you have severe, or very severe or advanced, COPD, you don't have to stay at home all the time.
- There is a lot you can do to stay healthy and enjoy your life.

Ask yourself this:

Am I connected with a pulmonary rehabilitation program, local breathing support group, or online COPD community?

This week:

- If you're not connected with one of the above, consider it. The COPD Foundation hosts COPD360social, an online social community. www.copdfoundation.org/COPD360social/Community/Activity-Feed.aspx
- If you already are connected to one of the above, log on or tell your support group friends that you are thankful for them, then do something to help someone.

September – Week 1

Harmonica Playing with COPD

"Music's the medicine of the mind."

– John A. Logan

Always consult your physician before starting any new breathing-related activity. This chapter is for information only and not intended as medical advice.

If you have COPD you might feel that taking on something new would be difficult and overwhelming. What about learning to play a musical instrument, especially one that requires breathing? You may be thinking, "I don't feel up to learning something new, I don't see the point in playing music, and I barely have enough breath to get through my day, let alone spend my breath on that!" But, before you write this off completely, let's take a few minutes to look at harmonica playing with COPD.

Harmonica playing for individuals with COPD and other chronic lung diseases has been in existence for some time. The harmonica is played when you blow (exhale) and draw (inhale) through openings on the instrument. As you do this the air moves through the reeds of the harmonica and musical notes are created. When you exhale into a harmonica you are breathing against a slight resistance, helping you get some of the same benefits that you get with pursed-lips breathing.

We talked about pursed-lips breathing in chapter July – Week 1, but here's a quick review. Doing pursed-lips breathing helps you slow your breathing down and be in better control of your breathing. Breathing against a slight resistance causes "back pressure" inside your airways, keeping them open longer. This helps your lungs get rid of more stale, trapped air. Pursed-lips breathing helps increase the amount of time you can exercise or perform an activity. It also improves the exchange of oxygen and carbon dioxide.

We talked about diaphragmatic breathing in chapter July – Week 2. The diaphragm is a large muscle that is meant to do most of the work of breathing. When you play the harmonica, you are exercising your diaphragm while drawing air in and blowing air out. Because the diaphragm is a muscle, it can be exercised and sometimes get stronger.

In addition to exercising the diaphragm, playing the harmonica can also help strengthen the muscles between your ribs, as well as some in your abdomen (belly). When these muscles are stronger, you may have a more effective cough and clear your lungs more easily. Breathing properly while you play the harmonica may also help improve your posture.

Okay, that sounds great. But let's face it, we all like to do things we enjoy. Here are some other benefits. Playing the harmonica can:

- Help you focus on learning a new skill.
- Encourage you to have more patience and purpose.
- Help you get out and socialize and be an active part of a group.
- Give you a sense of accomplishment.
- Be enjoyable and fun.

At this time there have been no studies done that are significant enough to prove that harmonica playing with COPD improves lung function. But people who play the harmonica, especially those who are part of a harmonica group, report many benefits. Here are some benefits described by individuals with COPD and other chronic lung diseases after participating in one of the COPD Foundation's *Harmonicas for Health** pilot programs. Again, these benefits are reported by the harmonica players themselves – they have not been proven as part of any research study.

*Please note that it is not necessary to be part of a COPD Foundation Harmonicas for Health program to have these benefits. Know that playing the harmonica, especially in a group setting with peers who have chronic lung disease, can be of great value to those who play.

60 new harmonica players were asked to complete this sentence: *Since I've been playing the harmonica, I feel I have:*
(The number indicates the percent of people in that group that reported each benefit.)

- Less shortness of breath 30%
- More energy 15%
- Better ability to cough up mucus 27%
- Been in more control of my breathing 48%
- Been more active 20%
- Felt less stress 47%
- Had less depression 29%
- Been more social 42%
- More confidence in myself 32%
- An improved quality of life 23%

Here, three respiratory therapists tell us about their *Harmonicas for Health* programs. Each program is unique when it comes to where, when, and in what setting it takes place. But all these programs have the most important things in common – they all bring people together to make music with new friends, have fun, and think about their breathing in a new and refreshing way.

The quotes you see are from participants in the *Harmonicas for Health* pilot programs.

Stacey Blank, BTPS, RRT
Maryland

We have a small but committed breathing support group. Members of the group love playing the harmonica! They talk a lot and laugh a lot. It's easy to see that they are relaxing and enjoying each other's company. The first time we used a metronome app on my phone to help keep time, this led to discussions about smart phones, health apps, and how healthcare is changing. Leading a harmonica group is such a good way to open up dialogue between the members! Every other month we focus on exercise and harmonicas. We start out with breathing exercises via the harmonica, then progress to basic songs, and then more difficult ones. We also introduce pulmonary rehabilitation patients to harmonicas and encourage them to come to our breathing support group meetings to continue playing. One of our members has a lot of mucus and great difficulty with airway clearance. He says that playing the harmonica helps him cough up mucus as well as some of his other therapies!

"This gives me the chance to meet other people, not take myself so seriously, have a good laugh, and achieve a goal!"

Darcy Ellefson, RRT AE-C
South Dakota

After several months of playing the harmonica, one of the men in my group reported that he had been to his pulmonologist. The doctor asked his patient if he had been doing anything different for his lungs because he had improved since his last appointment. The gentleman proudly said, 'I play my harmonica every day.' His doctor was quite impressed! To be honest, this gentleman is not a very good harmonica player, but that doesn't matter. He still benefits from the lung exercise the harmonica gives him but more importantly, he benefits from the socialization, laughs, and comradery every week with his fellow harmonica players. A lady in the group who learned how to play the harmonica in pulmonary rehab, occasionally plays in her small-town church during Sunday service. She also plays in the local nursing home for the residents as they sing along.

"Playing the harmonica helps my breathing without my thinking about it, and it's fun."

Dave P. Folds III, VHA CM
Florida

At first, I wasn't sure what to expect. I was somewhat cautious. After all, good medicine is based on solid evidence from either a big study or numerous small studies with same or similar results.

We started with five vets in our first class, four men (one was 92 years old, the others in their middle 70's) and a woman who was 69. This lady came to the first class with a small oxygen tank on a cart. By the third class she was leaving her oxygen in the car as she walked to class. All the fellas made similar improvements in their breathing.* They were walking more and really enjoyed the comradeship of others in the class. We have since grown to as many as 16 people in one class which might be too many. Twelve people in a class seems to be the best.

*These results are not typical for people with COPD who participate in harmonica playing. This particular improvement was likely the result of using more effective breathing patterns, better posture, and overall adherence to the individuals' medical regimens.

> *"I'm feeling confident and more aware of my*
> *breathing – overall feeling better about myself."*

Our Public Affairs office heard of the progress and posted an article on Facebook and our local VA webpage. Before we knew it, our office was deluged with requests. A local college NPR radio program did a story on the class and then National Public Radio ran the story in some national markets. As a result, some other VA hospitals have begun to pick up the *Harmonicas for Health* program.

This is the most fun I have had in 25 years working in healthcare. Also, this is the most I've seen people get involved in their own care. *Harmonicas for Health* is a true gift to the COPD population.

COPD is a progressive, sometimes debilitating, and currently incurable disorder often leading to a decline in overall health and a life of isolation and despair. But it doesn't have to be that way! With the right help and support, people with COPD can live a long time, not only surviving – but thriving – with COPD. Playing the harmonica can help.

Your Turn

Key points, or…If you don't remember anything else from this chapter, remember this:

- Harmonica playing for people with COPD does not claim to improve lung function numbers.
- Harmonica playing for people with COPD can, however, help exercise the lungs and be enjoyable and fun.

Ask yourself this:

Should I consider learning how to play the harmonica?

This week:

Look up harmonica playing with COPD on the internet and/or talk with a respiratory health professional about it.

Here's more help:

The COPD Foundation offers the first nationwide harmonica program created especially for individuals with COPD and other chronic lung diseases. Development of the *Harmonicas for Health* program was a collaboration of respiratory health educators, pulmonary physicians, and respiratory therapists with decades of experience leading harmonica groups. http://www.copdfoundation.org/HarmonicasforHealth

September – Week 2

Have I Got a Cure for You! Understanding Alternative Treatments for COPD

"Only a fool tests the depth of the water with both feet."

~ African Proverb

As a respiratory therapist I'm often asked about alternative treatments for COPD such as herbs, vitamins, mechanical breathing aides, breathing techniques, body manipulation, massage, etc. Sometimes the advertising – especially the testimonials – sounds so convincing. To sort it all out, I talked with pulmonary expert, Dr. Robert "Sandy" Sandhaus, MD, PhD, FCCP of the National Jewish Center, the number one respiratory hospital* in the United States. Think of these expert answers the next time you're wondering if an alternative or additional treatment is right for you.

*Source: *National Jewish Health was ranked the #1 respiratory hospital in the U.S. for the 18th time by U.S. News & World Report in its 2019 Best Hospitals rankings.*

1. Whenever I hear about something other than a "traditional" medicine for COPD, my doctor tells me it's no good. C'mon, aren't the big drug

companies saying these new methods are no good just to keep us buying their products?

I think everyone wants to find ways to help or cure disease that are mild, "natural," and non-injurious. Because of this, there is a tendency to head toward alternative treatments, especially if more traditional therapies are either not working well for you or are causing side effects that seem worse than the disease.

The challenge is to know what works and what doesn't – for you – and choosing from among the hundreds of agents and claims of success.

The reason most doctors are much more comfortable with "traditional" medications and therapies is that they have been tested, evaluated, approved, and often retested over and over, to find the best doses and combinations. The initial source of these medications may well be an herb or other agent that might have been considered "alternative" in the past.

Other medications are based on a scientific understanding of disease mechanisms and actions. These two methods of discovering new drugs are well represented in COPD therapies. Still, COPD deaths have been rising and there are many individuals who still have severe symptoms in spite of regular use of traditional medications.

Given the above, it would be great to have a natural or herbal remedy one could take that would make their COPD significantly improve. One may exist somewhere. The question is how would we know? Alternative medications are not subjected to the traditional testing and retesting or study and re-study, that traditional medicines do.

In general, the success stories are either by word of mouth or by an "expert" trying to sell a product or program, often with dramatic claims of success. It seems unlikely that all the claims and stories are true, otherwise there would be a lot of cured COPD patients out there. So how do you choose? I just don't have an answer to that question.

In addition, there is a growing appreciation that some herbal or alternative medications can actually lead to quite significant side effects and, especially, dangerous interactions with other medications, whether traditional or alternative.

Finally, there is the dubious question of whether docs and drug companies actually know how to cure COPD but won't do it because they want their patients to keep coming back to provide income, or the drug companies just want to sell their medications. Certainly, drug companies do want to make money! But, speaking as a doctor who treats patients with COPD every day, if I could prescribe or recommend a medication that cured COPD, I would be the happiest doctor in the world.

2. What's wrong with using herbal remedies for pulmonary problems? Herbs are natural so they can't hurt me, isn't that right?

Herbs may be just fine. Nevertheless, the fact that something is an herb doesn't guarantee it is either safe or effective. As mentioned above, herbs can interact with other medications, both natural and traditional. Don't forget that most poisons were initially isolated from plants and herbs.

3. What about some breathing methods offered in seminars? They come from countries other than the United States. Are we, in the United States, just being self-centered, believing that only we have all the answers?

Breathing exercise and training have an important place in many pulmonary diseases, especially COPD. Many pulmonary rehabilitation programs incorporate a variety of methods into their instruction. Several studies have evaluated non-traditional breathing methods such as Yoga and Buteyko as an adjunct to COPD therapy. The studies have shown mixed results.

In part, this appears to be due to the fact that some methods, like Buteyko, have no standardized methodology and often include components that are educational and nutritional. While studies have shown less bronchodilator usage in patients instructed in some form of Buteyko, there has been no change in their lung function or exercise tolerance. Often the control group also has a strong positive response, although not as dramatic as the treatment group, suggesting that just getting into a program that takes an interest in your overall health is beneficial to a COPD patient.

4. I've seen some books that talk about COPD being curable. In just one quick search I found several articles that came up when I entered "COPD Cure."

I know that many sites/individuals claim they have done scientific studies to prove their program's effectiveness – things like sheep stem cells injected into the lungs in a clinic, or oxidant or antioxidant medications that allow the lung to repair its damage.

Not only do these therapies and studies not stand up to close evaluation, they may well be quite harmful to those taking them. Finally, when you actually contact the centers offering these cures, you find that many want a substantial, up-front cash payment. This should make you very suspicious. *See the Added Insight at the end of this chapter for more on stem cell therapy.*

5. What about Vitamin "O" or oxygen drops to improve your oxygen levels? I got something in the mail with testimonials about how this helps people breathe better and I know someone personally who says he thinks it helps.

One of the biggest scams in the alternative medication arena, centers on the promotion of oxygen preparations taken by mouth. Whether drinks or drops or pills or capsules, there is no true scientific evidence of benefit and the rationale behind them is highly suspect – some may even do physical harm (in addition to the damage to your wallet).

First, there is no evidence that there is any significant uptake of oxygen in the stomach or intestines, even if you could deliver oxygen there. The air sacs in the lungs are microscopically thin so oxygen can cross their specialized membrane to move from the lungs into the blood. The stomach and intestines have no such apparatus to allow for the easy passage of oxygen.

Second, the ways that these products deliver "oxygen" is highly suspect. Among the products claiming to provide increased oxygen, the delivery approaches include making the solution high in dissolved oxygen, addition of "oxygen generating" chemicals, and addition of minerals that have oxygen in their formula. The most common mineral on earth, silicon dioxide (sand), has two oxygen molecules in its formula but that doesn't mean it will deliver oxygen to your body – so don't eat it!

You can make a solution that has extra oxygen dissolved in it by bubbling oxygen through it, especially at high pressure. But after you've done that if you leave the solution exposed to air, it will lose all that extra oxygen in a matter of minutes. The most common chemical used as an oxygen generate is hydrogen peroxide, a chemical well known as a potent oxidant. Sure, it generates oxygen, but a very caustic, free-radical type.

The claims advertised for these oxygen liquids include, in addition to increasing the oxygen in your blood, the ability to kill cancer cells, bacterial viruses, and toxins. Most web sites advertising these products make claims that bacteria, germs, and cancer cells can't survive when there is plenty of oxygen around. Actually, most cancer cells and bacteria LOVE oxygen and will grow more vigorously in its presence.

So why are there people who swear by these products? Probably because there are a certain number of people who will feel better with any new therapy. There is the "placebo effect" as one explanation. Another is that some people feel better when they take responsibility for their own care. Finally, there are some who would have started feeling better anyway and taking this medication coincided with their better health.

This is one class of alternative therapies I'd recommend avoiding.

6. What about Omega-3 Fatty Acids? I've been hearing more about it helping people with pulmonary disease. Mary Pierce (lady with Alpha-1 and recipient of a highly successful double-lung transplant) talked about it years ago and now I'm hearing that they really are helpful in pulmonary disease – or is this more related to prevention?

Omega-3 Fatty Acids are a necessary dietary component and there is growing evidence of its anti-inflammatory and other beneficial effects. Its actual role in lung disease is unclear at this time but, since COPD and many other lung diseases have inflammation as a prominent component, this may well prove an effective adjunctive therapy. Besides, I'd never disagree with Mary Pierce!

Added Insight

Stem cell therapy

This is a brief summary of the COPD Foundation's position on autologous (from a patient's own body) stem cell therapy. The entire position paper, "Autologous [from a patient's own body] Stem Cell Therapy is not Recommended for the Treatment of COPD" can be found at www.copdfoundation.org.

Stem cells are relatively immature or undifferentiated cells (that means they can become lots of different kinds of things from blood cells to lung cells to muscle cells) that are found within a variety of organs, including the lungs, or more distant sites (particularly the bone marrow) in even more undifferentiated forms. Their role is not yet fully understood, but there is some evidence that these cells can participate in the repair process following an injury.

The observation that stem cells taken from one's own body – autologous stem cells – might possess the ability to repair injured tissues, has given hope that stem cells may be used to restore normal function to severely damaged organs, including the lungs. What is not yet understood is which cells are most appropriate for this purpose, or how to direct those cells to repair and restore normal function, particularly in an organ as complex as the lung.

Clinics in and outside of the United States take autologous stem cells from one body tissue, usually fat tissue, and process these cells to enrich their number. Reinjection of these cells into the blood stream or via inhalation provides hope that they will stick to the target organ, such as the lung.

Claims of improvement and cure are implied, but are not stated clearly, at least by clinics operating within the United States. Instead, these clinics rely on personal testimonials from patients who have had this type of therapy. None claim direct scientific proof of the effectiveness of this therapy, in fact they note that the Food and Drug Administration (FDA) has not approved this type of therapy to treat lung diseases such as COPD.

Autologous stem cell therapy is not currently recommended for the treatment of COPD. Instead, participation in clinical trials that test the development and potential benefit of this technique is strongly encouraged.

There are many clinical trials ongoing worldwide on the use of stem cell therapy in the treatment of a wide variety of diseases. Over 4,000 such trials are listed within the United States (www.clinical-trials.gov). At least ten studies are actively recruiting people to test this therapy in the management of COPD.

Scientific proof of the effectiveness of these COPD treatments currently in use has come from painstaking research, particularly in the form of well-designed clinical trials.

None of these COPD trials are at the phase-3 level (working on definitively proving their effectiveness in people with COPD). Rather, they are focusing on safety and testing, like the best ways to give the cells, which cells to give, and how much to give. Again, it is this type of careful, step-by-step research that can add to our knowledge of how to best treat COPD and how to use stem cell therapy to manage this disease.

It is understandable that people who are desperate might seek any means of improvement or hope of a cure for their condition, even if unproven. Patient testimonials only, are not proof of effectiveness and safety of a medication or other therapy. These testimonials based on patient experience can be misleading to those who are seeking treatment of their COPD.

Autologous stem cell therapy may someday fulfill the promise of restoring or fixing damaged lung tissue, or provide a cure for COPD, but there is little evidence that this will happen within the foreseeable future. The COPD Foundation strongly recommends against the use of autologous stem cell therapy in the treatment of COPD or other lung disease, until there is more rigorous scientific and medical proof of its effectiveness. In contrast, the COPD Foundation strongly encourages support for further research and well-designed clinical trials to further develop this therapeutic approach.

Your Turn

Key points, or…if you don't remember anything else from this chapter, remember this:

- You should not believe everything you read or hear about new treatments for COPD.
- New, untraditional therapies are often put into practice before they are widely tested.
- Unscrupulous people tend to target people who are desperate for relief from symptoms.

Ask yourself this:

Have the medications and therapies I take for my COPD been proven safe and effective?

This week:

If you currently take, or are considering beginning to take, an alternative therapy, ask your doctor if it is safe and effective.

September – Week 3

Facing Fall - Preventing Exacerbations and When to Call the Doctor

To our friends in the southern hemisphere, this week, read May – Week 3: Gardening and Yardwork

"An ounce of prevention is worth a pound of cure."

~ Benjamin Franklin

The voice of the ER unit secretary came across my pager. "Stat neb treatment and ABG's in the emergency room – Stat neb treatment and ABG's in the emergency room."

It was 10:00pm on a cool fall night, the start of flu season. I walked into ER room six to find Steve, a man in his mid-60's, sitting on the edge of the gurney, leaning forward, coughing hard, and struggling to breathe. I took a sample of arterial blood to test his oxygen and carbon dioxide levels and put it on ice. I'd run the sample later, but right now the most important thing was to give Steve some relief. I handed him a hand-held nebulizer, already misting with a medicine to open his lungs. He put it to his mouth and breathed it in.

I patted his shoulder and said, "Not doing too well tonight, are you? Have you been sick for a while?"

"Nope. I was… fine until… tonight. This came… out of… nowhere."

"Hmmmm…" I said. "Steve, I have a few questions for you. Go ahead and breathe in your medication and just nod to say 'yes' or shake your head to answer 'no.' Okay?"

Steve nodded.

"Have you been coughing any more than usual over the last few days?"

Taking deeper breaths now and looking a bit more comfortable, Steve nodded.

"Have you been coughing anything up?"

Again, he nodded.

"Was it any different than usual? Did it have color to it? Was it thick and sticky?"

Steve gave me kind of a dirty look, like I'd asked a weird, unwanted question, one to those outside the respiratory world. It probably was. Then he said, "Come to think of it…I've been coughing up green stuff…for about a week."

Steve was not a stupid man, nor was he careless. He had recently quit smoking and generally took pretty good care of himself, but he had no idea – nobody ever told him – that for him, a person with COPD, a change in cough and a change in the color of mucus is just one major early warning sign of lung infection. If Steve had only known what to watch for and sought help at the first sign of trouble, he'd probably be at home right now, able to make it through this infection with a day or two off work and resting at home. Instead, he was in the ER, facing a two or three-day hospital stay and a week off of work.

One of the biggest concerns for a person with COPD is becoming sick, having an acute exacerbation (a period of worsened symptoms, usually due a respiratory infection), getting pneumonia, going downhill and losing ground, never fully recovering to where they were.

As a person with COPD, your job is to be on the look-out for early warning signs of acute exacerbation. A cold or flu germ that is a mere inconvenience to somebody with normal healthy lungs can become a major problem for you, possibly leading to something very serious. But there are things you can do to stave off an acute exacerbation of COPD. This is not to say you'll be completely successful each and every time, but if you know what to avoid and what signs to watch for, you'll be in a much better position to minimize illness and keep on living your life.

Avoiding germs

Here are just a few of the many things you can do to avoid picking up nasty bugs. I'm sure you can think of others that work well for you.

- Get your flu shot every fall.
- Ask your doctor about a pneumonia shot, which type is best for you and how long it should be before you get another pneumonia shot, if at all.
- Wash your hands with warm water and mild soap. Wash for fifteen seconds, the time it takes to sing "Twinkle, Twinkle Little Star." (You don't have to sing aloud!)
- Use your own pen. Do you really want to touch the pen that everybody uses at the bank – or worse, the pharmacy or doctor's office? If you have to use the "pen" they use to sign on the screen, use hand sanitizer immediately after touching it.
- If you can't wipe off the handle on the grocery cart, wear lightweight gloves or cover the handle with a disposable fruit and vegetable bag as you shop.
- Carry hand sanitizer with you and use it when you can't wash.

Develop an action plan with your doctor

Work in partnership with your doctor to stay well. Make an appointment if you don't have one coming up soon. At this appointment, ask:

"When do you want me to call you?"

"Which early warning signs do you want to know about when I notice them?"

"When I call your office, how will your staff know that I'm more likely than many of your other patients to get really sick?"

Know what to watch for

Knowing early warning signs cannot only help you stay healthy, at home, and independent, but it can even save your life! Here are some early warning signs of acute exacerbation for people with COPD. Show this list to your doctor and ask if there are any other early warning signs, specific to you and your situation, that he or she suggests you watch for.

- A change in your cough – are you coughing more, less, or is it different than your usual?
- A change in the amount or color in your mucus. Is it yellow, green, or bloody? Your mucus should be clear or white.
- If you have a pulse oximeter at home, are your O_2 sats (oxygen saturations) lower than usual?
- Have you just had a sudden weight gain such as three to five pounds overnight?
- Do you have swelling in your ankles or feet? Here's a tip: Gently press the tip of your finger into the skin around your ankles and feet. Does it leave a dent? It shouldn't. If it does, call your doctor.
- Do you have morning dizziness, confusion, or a headache

that doesn't go away with commonly used over-the-counter pain medications?

- Is your heart rate faster than usual (60-100 is normal, with each person having their own "normal"). Know your normal resting heart rate.
- Your urine should be pale yellow and clear with no odor. If it is darker than usual, cloudy, or with a foul odor, you might have a urinary tract infection.
- Do you have a fever?
- Are you unusually tired?
- Do you have joint or muscle aches that are unusual for you?

Don't spend this fall and winter on the edge of a COPD exacerbation! If you catch early warning signs and work in partnership with your doctor, you have a much better chance at stopping an infection in its tracks so you can stay well, stay home, and keep on living your life.

Your Turn

Key points, or...if you don't remember anything else from this chapter, remember this:

- Do what you can to avoid lung infections.
- Know the early warning signs of acute exacerbation.
- Develop an action plan with your doctor about when to call and how to make sure the office staff pays attention.

Ask yourself this:

Do I know my early warning signs of acute exacerbation?

This week:

Make an appointment with your doctor for a flu shot, and to talk about how you can stay healthy this fall and winter.

Here's more help:

The *My COPD Action Plan* and the *Report Exacerbations* card are available from the COPD Foundation as a free download. www. copdfoundation.org/Learn-More/Educational-Materials-Resources/ Downloads-Library.aspx

September – Week 4

Cough and Airway Clearance

"You gotta do what you gotta do."

~ Sylvester Stallone

Secretions. Phlegm. Sputum. Mucus. Yuck! Whatever you call it, that junk in your lungs is yet another part of having COPD that's not all that much fun. Still, it's one of those things that as a person with COPD, you just have to deal with – and if you learn what to expect and how to handle it, you'll breathe easier.

What's the role and function of sputum in the lungs?

Before we talk about getting rid of mucus, we need to understand why we have it in the first place. The lungs provide protection against foreign substances entering the body by stopping unwanted particles and trapping them before they get too deep into your lungs.

The bronchial airways (tubes in your lungs that the air goes through) inside your lungs are lined with a thin layer of mucus. Just underneath this mucus are cilia, millions of tiny little hair-like structures. The cilia move like a wave to help propel the mucus upward – carrying with it trapped dust, bacteria, and other substances – where they can be coughed out. This is how your lungs keep themselves clean. Mucus also acts to humidify the air you breathe. As your air makes its way through your bronchial airways, it passes over the mucus, picking up moisture.

Dirty lungs

We know that the cilia, the little sweepers in your airways, help keep your lungs clean. But cigarette smoke and other irritants in our environment can destroy or paralyze them. This causes the cilia to stop working and thus, your lungs are not able to clean themselves as they should. Along with this the bronchial airways can become chronically (all the time) or acutely (suddenly and temporarily) inflamed (swollen). As a result, the mucus in your airways can become thicker and stickier.

With the loss of your normal cleaning mechanism, as well as a tendency towards thicker, stickier secretions and swollen airways, you can see why breathing with COPD can be so hard! With all this going on, your lungs have to figure out another way to get rid of excess mucus and that's why you may have a frequent, productive cough. If you cough on most days, producing mucus even when you do not have an acute infection, you probably have chronic bronchitis. Talk with your doctor about this at your next appointment.

Yes, all this sticky mucus can make it hard to breathe, but there's another reason why it's important to keep your lungs clear. You need to keep your lungs as clear – and as healthy – as possible because if too much mucus stays in your lungs, it can cause ongoing inflammation, which can lead to further lung damage, and more coughing, making you tired and even more breathless.

What can I do to keep my lungs clear?

- Drink two quarts of water a day if okay with your doctor.
- Take an expectorant or mucolytic (a medication that helps you cough up mucus). This can be ordered by your doctor,

or you can take a non-prescription expectorant if your doctor says it's okay.

- Use proper cough techniques. Sit up straight but bending slightly forward supporting your elbows. A straight chair with armrests works well.
- If possible, do not lie down when coughing. Coughing is much more effective when you're sitting up.
- Use the huff cough technique. Ask a respiratory therapist to show you.
- Ask your doctor if percussion and postural drainage might help. If so, a respiratory therapist can train your family member or caregiver how to give you this therapy.
- Use an airway clearance device if directed (see below).
- Take time for your bronchial hygiene each day, just as you take time to wash your face or brush your teeth.

Bronchiectasis and Nontuberculous Mycobacteria (NTM) lung disease

Bronchiectasis is a chronic lung disease in which the bronchial airways become widened, scarred, and inflamed. In bronchiectasis, like some types of COPD, the cilia don't work normally. This can cause mucus to pool in the bronchial airways, allowing bacteria to grow, resulting in an increased number of lung infections. Causes of bronchiectasis include injury from foods and liquids getting into the lungs, immune deficiencies, inflammatory diseases, and genetically inherited disorders.

Another cause of bronchiectasis is repeated lung infections, sometimes caused by specific bacteria. One such bacteria is NTM, a naturally occurring bacteria found in soil and water. It is not harmful to most people but can cause NTM lung disease in people with COPD, bronchiectasis, asthma, and other chronic disorders. It's important to know, however, that just because you may have COPD or another chronic lung problem, that doesn't mean that you will get NTM lung disease.

Here's a report on Mucus Clearance Devices contributed by Richard D. Martin, the Editor of *COPD-NEWS*. Thank you to Richard for granting his permission to include this information.

In some cases, our doctors or respiratory therapists might recommend we use a hand-held mechanism that loosens the mucus to make it easier to cough out. These small devices vibrate when we breathe into them and are known by various names, such as "percussive airway devices," or "vibratory positive expiratory pressure (PEP) devices." They use vibrations and air pressure to reduce the thickness of mucus. Although the devices are used more commonly for individuals with cystic fibrosis and bronchiectasis, they are also used to help those of us with COPD who have difficulty getting rid of mucus.

There are a number of brands on the market. They all require a prescription. *(Author's note: Device brand names are included in this chapter so you can learn about them. This is not intended as a promotion.)* The most commonly recognized brands are Acapella, Flutter, Lung Flute, and Quake, although there are others. Your doctor or respiratory therapist may recommend a particular brand for a specific reason. In some cases, they actually keep a small supply on hand and dispense them directly to patients. It pays, however, to be familiar with the major brands.

If you are prescribed a device be sure to have a respiratory therapist teach you how to use it properly. It may seem simple, but there is more to it than just blowing into them!

If you cannot locate information on a device, do an internet search using the name or ask your respiratory health professional.

Acapella®

This device shakes your mucus loose when you blow into it. It must be dialed to the proper setting by someone who is trained it is in use. It will work if you are laying down. Visit the manufacturer's web site at: http://tinyurl.com/33tfgh

Flutter®

The Flutter works in a similar way, but you must be sitting or standing up straight to use it. You can read about this device on the manufacturer's web site: https://medinstrum.com/flutter-mucus-clearance-device/

Lung Flute®

The Flute creates vibrations to loosen the mucus by passing air over a reed. The device includes a six-month supply of reeds. An additional six-month supply must be purchased. You can order them directly (prescription needed) from the manufacturer at: http://tinyurl.com/29epc7y

Quake®

For more information about the Quake, visit the manufacturer's web site:
http://thayermedical.com/products/quake/

Added Insight

When Coughing is Too Distasteful – an article by Dr. Francis Adams

A lifetime of suppression leads to infection – and a very unladylike treatment for Lady Windermere Syndrome.

Excerpted from the story by Francis V. Adams, special to The Los Angeles Times, March 26, 2007.

Coughing was a no-no for a proper lady.

I saw another Lady Windermere the other day. Over the years I have seen several patients who could have borne this name. The character, who originated in Oscar Wilde's play, "Lady Windermere's Fan" was a fastidious woman who would become a symbol of the Victorian era, an age when women wouldn't do *anything* they thought vulgar, such as spitting.

My first Lady Windermere was Agatha. I met her not long after I finished my training in pulmonary disease and opened my private practice. I glimpsed her in the waiting room as I picked up her chart. As she sat in my office, I inquired as to what had brought her, and she went on to describe an unrelenting cough she'd had for nearly ten years. During the interview, she coughed fitfully but would not expectorate.

Agatha was 63, very thin, almost skeletal, with high cheekbones, thin lips and a straight nose. She held a tiny lace handkerchief in her left hand and covered her mouth as she coughed.

I proceeded to take Agatha's medical history. She had been in good health except for her chest problems, which she described as frequent colds that always settled in her chest. Agatha had been hospitalized twice for pneumonia. Her lung sounds were a bit quieter than normal, but I did not detect any congestion. I proceeded to take an X-ray, which showed that the air passages in the middle sections were thicker than normal.

We sat in my office and I told her that it would help if she could bring up some sputum for the lab to analyze for infection. I also explained that additional X-rays would be helpful.

Agatha said that she was used to having X-rays but doubted if she would be able to produce a sample of her sputum. Just then she coughed again, and I noted that she seemed to be trying to suppress her effort.

I told her that I had a few tricks for getting people to cough up. I took Agatha into another room and introduced her to a nebulizer, a simple machine that creates an aerosol mist by forcing air through a solution. I placed saline into the machine, attached some tubing, turned on the power and saw a steam-like vapor emitted.

I asked her to breathe the mist for ten minutes and placed a sputum cup on the counter next to the nebulizer. When I returned to the room, I saw that the cup was still empty. I placed more saline into the machine and asked her to try again. After the second treatment, Agatha coughed and produced a tiny bit of yellow sputum. The sputum sample was sent off to the lab and her X-rays scheduled. I explained that I hoped to have the results of both tests in a few days.

Agatha's X-rays showed that there was evidence of old and new infection in the middle sections of both lungs. The bronchial tubes in both areas had been damaged causing them to dilate and become congested with mucus, a condition known as bronchiectasis. Bronchiectasis is usually produced by an untreated lung infection. In many of my elderly patients of that time, the infection had occurred in childhood when antibiotics were not yet available.

The culture of the tiny piece of expectorated sputum yielded an organism known as mycobacterium avium intracellulare. This is a bacterium that lives in nature and can be found in the soil or water. Agatha had no history of childhood infection, so I wondered if the over-fastidiousness that kept her from clearing secretions had in fact promoted the development of her condition. I proceeded to outline a course of treatment that would include three antibiotics over a period of one-and-a-half years. I also placed her on an expectorant and arranged for a physical therapist to cup and clap her chest twice a week, hoping to help clear her air passages. Despite these efforts, my patient's cough did not produce sputum.

During the long course of Agatha's treatment, I saw two more women who bore not only a physical resemblance to her but also the identical illness. Irene was 68, a teacher with a widow's peak, and Constance was 60, a librarian. Both had similar X-ray changes as Agatha, and their sputum, which I obtained with great difficulty, also yielded the same organism. All three women were cooperative, intelligent, and easy to work with, but I became increasingly frustrated by their failure to clear their lungs despite the many maneuvers that I put them through.

After my third case, I consulted my colleagues and the medical literature, and found that I was not alone. Other doctors were seeing similar patients. In 1992, fifteen years after I first met Agatha, two radiologists published a report of "The Lady Windermere Syndrome." They had observed six women with the same characteristics as my patients. The authors noted that the middle portions of the lungs extend outward toward the front of the chest and require vigorous coughing for clearance of secretions. They concluded that mycobacterial infection had occurred in these overly fastidious women due to voluntary suppression of cough.

Agatha's infection was not cured by years of treatment but did improve. I continue to see a few women each year with the same striking features and pride myself on making the correct diagnosis simply from observing their appearance and hearing their cough before they are seated in my office.

A few of these delicate women have found me through Internet searches so that after introducing myself to one of these ladies recently, she replied: "And you may call me Lady Windermere."

Your Turn

Key points, or…if you don't remember anything else from this chapter, remember this:

- Lungs have a built-in cleaning system that can be disabled with COPD.
- It's important to do all you can to keep your lungs clear, not only for good health now, but to protect your lungs from further damage.
- There are many things you can do to help clear your lungs.

Ask yourself this:

Do I cough every day?

Do I bring up mucus?

Do I have trouble bringing up mucus, feeling like it's "stuck?"

This week:

If you answer "yes" to any of the three questions above, make sure you're taking all the steps in the section of this chapter, "What Can I Do to Keep My Lungs Clear?" Consider asking your healthcare provider if you might have bronchiectasis.

At the Bronchiectasis and NTM initiative, www.BronchiectasisnandNTMinitiative.org, you'll find BronchandNTM360social, a vibrant online community, educational information and materials, and information on research programs such as the Bronchiectasis and NTM Research Registry.

September – Week 5

Denial

"The worst lies are the lies we tell ourselves."

~ Richard Bach

When I was doing research for my first book, interviewing people with COPD – people from all walks of life, of all ages, from all over the country – I found that without exception there was one common thread connecting every story. Denial. Let's be honest, nobody wants to have an incurable, progressive disease, especially one that may have been brought on by a particular behavior. We're all human and we like to think of ourselves as being active and healthy. So of course, denial is extremely common in COPD.

This book is about COPD, and I am assuming that you, the reader, already know – or strongly suspect – that you have this disease. But, in this chapter we're going to turn the clock back and talk about that period of time, most likely a period of years, in which you didn't know you had COPD. A time when you first, but barely, noticed shortness of breath. And we're going to retrace your steps all the way up to that pivotal moment or event when finally, it was undeniable.

Small changes – what changes?

We're all getting older, and along with advancing age we can expect to slow down. Becoming short of breath is probably one of the most common small changes we experience – and one of the easiest to pass over as insignificant.

Cheri Register, author of _The Chronic Illness Experience,_ has a non-pulmonary related chronic disease, but we can learn a lot from her. She says, "The first challenge any illness poses is in deciding just when you are sick enough to worry about it. Often the initial problems are not that great a departure from your usual state of health. As annoying as they might be, you may be tempted to dismiss them, unless they are known to be danger signals, like the [more well-known] 'warning signs of cancer.' Everyone has aches and pains, after all, and most of them subside on their own. For fear of being called hypochondriacs, many of us would rather wait out the discomfort than risk seeming excessively alarmed."

Gradual changes – or – "maybe if I just ignore it, it'll go away."

When I asked Mary Pierce (see chapter April – Week 1) if she thought her husband, Todd, knew that something was wrong, Mary answered, "He says he didn't. When people later on asked him, 'Didn't you know that something was going on?' He answered, 'Well, I knew she was losing a lot of weight, but it just happened so gradually, I never noticed [the increasing shortness of breath].' Again, he was making all the little incremental adjustments along the way."

Cheri Register says, "It is not so much fear and denial as it is confusion and embarrassment that keep people out of the doctor's office in the early stages of illness. Having no clear sense of the boundaries that divide illness from health, we redraw our own as needed to keep ourselves functioning."

Whatever we call it, fear, denial, confusion, embarrassment, though COPD symptoms may temporarily subside, they eventually demand attention.

I was just fine until…

It's important to understand that in all but a few cases, by the time you seek help, your COPD has been progressing for quite some time, probably for years or even decades. A classic scenario is that the patient states that he or she was just fine until recently coming down with pneumonia. After some testing (chest X-ray, pulmonary function, arterial blood gas) and personal health history) it becomes abundantly clear to the doctor and, eventually to the patient, that lung disease has been present for many years. As the lungs become more and more compromised over time, they are less able to tolerate common insults such as colds and flu. What a shock to the person who feels they were fine until a recent illness is now told they have 30% lung function left (70% non-functional and beyond repair)!

Let's say that today you walk up to your car and notice a spot of rust. You never noticed it before. You're sure it wasn't there yesterday. But, do you think that until today the body of your car in that spot was perfectly intact, that it was solid, perfect metal and then, overnight, it broke through to form a rusty patch? No, you see the rust and realize then that it must have been coming on for quite a while.

An event – the tipping point

It's been said that denial is nature's way of giving us a good night's sleep. Maybe so, but this works only up to a point and especially with COPD, there comes a time when we can simply no longer deny the facts.

When I interviewed new patients coming into our pulmonary rehab program, one of the first questions I asked was when did they first notice their shortness of breath? Almost always, they tell me of a point in time, something they remember well, an event that tipped the scale to cause them to sit up and take notice. Made them notice that something was not only not right, but something was very wrong.

Cheri Register says, "We continue to tell these stories [of when the illness began] because it seems important to have a frame in which to contain the experience of chronic illness. The story needs a strong beginning because it has no structure otherwise. With chronic illness, there is no single climax, just the irregularly recurring ups and downs…Chronic illness does not fit the popular notion of how illness proceeds: 'You get sick, you go to the doctor and get some medicine, and wait to get better'…The best we can do to clear up the chaos in our lives is to look back and say, 'This is how it all began. This was when my life took an unfortunate turn.'"

Going way back

Back to the pulmonary rehab initial evaluation…as we talked, we'd often delve a bit deeper, and as we did the patient thought back to times *before* the turning point, saying, "Now that I think about it, I remember several years ago having some trouble keeping up. I figured I was getting older and out of shape, so I didn't think much of it."

Guilt and shame

Mary Pierce (a former smoker with Alpha-1 Antitrypsin Deficiency, genetically inherited COPD) said of her life before diagnosis, "The denial was definitely there…for a *long* time. It was like I was the only one that had *the secret*…a huge dark secret. The hiding. The shame. The guilt. You know, I'd seen other people with health problems worse than mine, things they didn't bring on themselves. I figured I'd shortened my life and all that. *I did it to myself*. At the time I didn't think it all the way through, but my reaction then was guilt, shame, embarrassment."

Relationships – with your family

Mary continues, "At least I felt that way, and I was hiding it from everybody. I was denying it and hiding it, and that was part of who I was. That alone prevented some of the close personal interactions. The wall was up, even with my family. The interactions became artificial. You know, pretending. I remember back when I could not do much of anything. I just didn't have the energy. I'd say, 'I can't. I've got to go do this or I've got to do that.' I'd just make an excuse somehow."

Relationships – with your doctor

Denial can also adversely affect your relationship with your healthcare provider. There can be no partnership in effective COPD management if the doctor is unaware of your breathing problems.

Consequently, without the right information, it's not possible to make informed decisions regarding life support, or "heroic" measures. The person with COPD needs to discuss advance directives issues with their family in order to make informed decisions together. The decisions must then be written down and placed where medical personnel and family can find them. Not doing so puts a burden on family members who are faced not only with making tough decisions in a time of crisis but need to make those decisions in light of a chronic diagnosis that to them – because of denial – seems so new. (See chapter October – Week 1, Advance Directives – Why You (and everybody) Should have a Living Will.)

In some cases, the diagnosis has been given, but understated by the doctor. Some patients are told by their doctor that they have a "little touch" of emphysema. This might even be considered denial on the part of the physician!

Mary Pierce says, "Those words 'a little touch' kind of puts the patient on notice that they don't have to worry about it. Hearing a wishy-washy diagnosis is like going into confessional and being forgiven."

Poor health management

With denial, there is no diagnosis. With no diagnosis there is no effective management, and one's overall health will only get worse. Denial of the existence of COPD can actually lead to a person having either less – or surprisingly more – treatment than needed. Treating each exacerbation as an isolated case, as just another "bout of bronchitis," can cause over-prescribing of antibiotics. Failure to treat COPD symptoms at all, on the other hand, denies the patient the opportunity to benefit from helpful medications, education, support, and exercise that can extend and improve the quality of life.

Does accepting a diagnosis mean I'm giving up and giving in?

Most importantly, just because you admit and accept the diagnosis of COPD doesn't mean you're giving in and giving up. Far from it! Acceptance gives you the permission and the *power* to acquire knowledge – knowledge that will arm you with weapons needed for the battle to fight your disease. (See chapter December – Week 1, War or Peace?)

Traveling that road from denial to acceptance and empowerment can be a long, painful journey. But when you know what you're facing, you can find help. With the support of knowledgeable respiratory health professionals, understanding peers, and a loving family, you can learn what works and what doesn't, what is achievable and what isn't, what is realistic and what is no longer safe to attempt. Finally, free from the grip of denial, you can gain control of your breathing with hope for the best possible life from that moment on.

Added Insight I

Tom's story

Meet Tom, a successful businessman with a drive to work hard and keep on going, no matter what. Here, in his own words, he gives us a glimpse of a fascinating timeline on his road to better breathing.

Let me start with a few flashbacks that seem to make sense now.

Age 31...I didn't have any problems. We were moving into a new house and my father, a healthy non-smoker of 71, was helping me carry things. After moving one particularly heavy desk a relatively short distance he was left gasping for air. I never thought much of this until recently. He was never diagnosed with a breathing disorder. He died of congestive heart failure four years later.

Age 39...I didn't have any problems. We were skiing at Alta. A big snow fell, and we were out first thing in the morning. I made a run to the bottom and fell in a heap. After catching my breath, I tried to get up, but the snow was too deep and I just wallowed around. It took me ten minutes of struggling and resting to finally get back to my feet. I thought I was going to faint.

Age 54...I didn't have any problems. I was at one of my daughter's high school basketball games...a championship at stake, a see-saw game with the crowd going wild. Suddenly I realized that after a cheer I had nothing left in my lungs. Gulp, gulp, a little air, please.

Age 61...I finally had a hunch that there was something wrong. I went skiing at Santa Fe and found that I could barely walk uphill more than 100 feet.

Age 63...I checked in with a pulmonologist who sent me over to the hospital for testing. Sure enough, I was operating with less than 40% of my expected lung capacity. He had suggestions about how I could manage my disease. But, of course, things got in the way and I put it off.

Age 64...I was standing in the grocery store gasping for breath...I had an infection, my lungs were full of liquid and I flat-out couldn't breathe.

So, I entered pulmonary rehabilitation. I guess my first thought when I was clearly told, and shown, that there was hard data that I had COPD was, "Well, let's get to work fixing this mess." I am a pretty hard-nosed realist and have spent my life in design and problem solving, so this was nothing new. I also reflected on the fact that I had a good idea of what it is that would kill me.

My first thought at starting pulmonary rehab was, "Wow, I'm in far better shape than everyone else here...I'm lucky to have this chance, and I better take it seriously and bust my butt to get in shape."

My daily life now is just as it has been these last ten years...except I am in rehab for two hours a week, I lift weights for two hours a week, I have learned how to do pursed-lips breathing, and I plan ahead and start breathing early when I know I'm headed for some stairs. You have to commit the time – and given the alternative – that should be easy.

I guess I was in denial for a long time. Certainly long enough! But now, after facing COPD head on, learning about it, and doing all I can to manage it, I have to tell you – my Quality of Life is better, and I have no doubt that my Quantity of Life will be better, too.

Added Insight II

Eileen's story

For several years I had known something was wrong. I was becoming more and more short of breath and kept telling myself that I had to quit smoking. It was difficult to do stairs and even walking any short distance was a chore. As far as I was concerned, I was a nurse and could treat myself. That idea almost proved fatal for me.

One day, throughout the day I was feeling more and more

breathless. Inhalers didn't help. I finally realized that I couldn't walk even one step without fighting for a breath. It was late at night before I told my daughter and had her call 9-1-1. As an independent person, and a nurse at that, I was mortified that I had to be carried down the stairs and into an ambulance! This kind of thing could happen to other people – but never to me!

By the time I arrived at the hospital, I was almost unconscious. I remember bits and pieces and being told that I needed to be on a ventilator. My daughter later told me, as did the doctor, that they didn't think I was going to make it. I was on a vent for three days and don't remember a thing. When I woke up, the pulmonary specialist came into my room and said: "You have COPD. If you quit smoking now, this will never happen again!"

But instead of listening to what he said, I hated him – as though it was his fault that I had to get the news. "Lousy bedside manner," I remember saying. Shortly after discharge, I was sneaking smokes and soon back at it full time.

After that I spent years minimizing my condition and pretending that I was just fine. A typical day would be, try to get out of bed and face the day knowing that even as I started my day, I was already exhausted. Many days I would call in to work and say I had a headache, or didn't sleep well the night before, and would be in late. Sometimes I could roll over and get another hour or two of sleep – but it never helped. After lying relatively still for several hours, my lungs would become 'stiff' and I would have to take several minutes with an inhaler at the side of my bed.

At some point I had to get up. Then to the bathroom. Then to the couch. More inhalers and pills and much coughing would leave me exhausted. Then it's time for a shower. I can't say how many times I called back in to work and stayed home just because I couldn't make myself get into the shower. Gather my things, get in, lather my hair, rinse it off, soap all over, rinse it off, shave, rinse it off – this all left me gasping for breath by the end. I would have to sit on the commode to finish wiping off. Then go to the bedroom and dress. Short of breath all the way. Take a break and then dry my hair. All the lifting of my arms and movement made me short of breath and almost not worth the trouble. Then take a rest. Then go to work.

Well, things just kept on going downhill. I became sick again and wound up in the hospital and on a ventilator again, this time for five days. My daughter was at my bedside night and day because again, no one thought I would live. But I did live and, under much protest went to pulmonary rehab. Even that wonderful gift did not stop my self-destructive behaviors. I couldn't stop smoking! I felt I was so needed at work, so I spent more time there than I did taking care of myself. I was a Director of Nursing and trying to balance a very hectic work life. As soon as I walked in the door, someone would confront me with issues...all day long this went on.

In my mind – I could do it all. But in the real world I couldn't. I let my work decline and my health declined right along with it. God forbid anyone should know how much I was suffering. I lied to work, to my doctors, to my family, and thought everything could go on status quo. But it couldn't.

I crashed and burned when I was hospitalized with cor pulmonale (right-sided heart failure due to COPD). Work said my performance was poor, and despite my valiant efforts, they were right. I knew my body was suffering and it was getting worse.   I finally resigned my position a month later. I was heartbroken. I had been a nurse for so long and loved it. My pride had suffered a devastating blow. Life would never be the same. I had been so proud to be a nurse, that's who and what I was, and now my life as I knew it seemed to be over for good.

Since then, reclaiming my life has meant I would have to take baby steps. First of all, I got serious about quitting smoking and I finally did it. I went back to pulmonary rehab and got serious about that too. Exercise wasn't a spectator sport anymore – it couldn't be if I were to survive. I went three times a week and even though I was a nurse, I gained so much knowledge along with energy, and more spirit than I've known in many years.

I got involved in an internet support group where I have an online family who is as important to me now as my own family. I try to reach out to others so that in helping others, I might find some meaning in my own life. Life is never certain, but it certainly is better now.

Your Turn

Key points, or…if you don't remember anything else from this chapter, remember this:

Getting past denial is an essential step in becoming empowered to live life to the fullest with COPD.

Ask yourself this:

Where am I in this process?

This week:

Write the timeline of your own journey from denial to empowerment.

Here's more help:

See Chapter May – Week 1 for the "Take Back Your Life" Framework.

Added Insight I - taken from *COPD and Denial: A Common Thread*, generously contributed by an anonymous COPD patient as part of an article written by Jane M. Martin, BA, LRT and published on COPDConnection.com. HealthCentral, 2010. All rights reserved. http://www.healthcentral.com/copd/c/19257/99878/denial-common-thread

October – Week 1

Advance Directives - Why You (and everybody) Should Have a Living Will

"Having the world's best idea will do you no good unless you act on it. People who want milk shouldn't sit on a stool in the middle of a field in hopes that a cow will back up to them."

~ Curtis Grant

Dr. Rajani, a tiny lady no more than five feet tall, shook my hand, looked me in the eye and said, "It's nice to meet you. Your father is a very sick man. His body is shutting down. Do you want us to put him on life support or should we make him a no code?

"Uh...can we watch him closely and see..."

She interrupted. "You have to make a decision. Soon."

This conversation was not exactly what I had in mind for my first meeting with this doc and certainly not the best way to begin a discussion on end of life issues!

My sister had called me the night before saying that Dad was in the hospital with shortness of breath but after getting settled in and being put on two liters of oxygen, he was feeling more comfortable and doing better. However, the next morning Mom called me at my hospital job in Michigan, saying, "Dad's taken a turn for the worse and they say he may not make it." Her voice wavered. "I need you here. You understand these things."

You see, as Dad got older, my sister and I had urged him to talk about what he would want done, medically, if he were to be unable to speak for himself. Stubborn Dutchman that he was (eighty years old at the time and more obstinate than ever), he refused. Now, here we were. Inaction on my father's part had put all of us – my mom, the doctors, my sister, and me – in this terrible, and most urgent, situation. Believe me, you don't want to find yourself in this position – and the good news is that you don't ever have to. Let's talk about advance directives, appointing a patient advocate, and living wills.

What is an advance directive?

An advance directive is a document saying what you would like done, medically, if you should ever be in a situation in which you're unable to speak for yourself. An advance directive allows you to make your own decisions – in advance – and by doing so have control over what happens to you, so others don't decide things for you. Telling your loved ones your wishes is a good first step, but it isn't enough. You must have it in writing.

What is a living will?

A living will is a legal document in which you can be specific regarding life-prolonging medical treatments. A living will should not be confused with a living trust, which has to do with holding and distributing your property and finances.

Who should have one?

Every adult should have a living will, even those who are young and healthy.

What is a durable power of attorney for health care?

This is the appointment of a patient advocate, one or two people you have chosen to speak for you, if you should ever be unable to speak for yourself. This could be a spouse, an adult child, or someone else you trust who is able, and willing, to take responsibility for carrying out your wishes. A durable power of attorney for health care cannot make decisions for you regarding your possessions, property, or money. It is for health-related issues only.

How do I start this discussion? Isn't it morbid and depressing? Will it scare my loved ones?

Nobody likes to think about dying or losing a loved one, but we are all going to die sometime and when we do, it should be on our own terms. Begin by assuring your loved ones that bringing up this subject doesn't mean you're planning to die anytime soon. Take a positive approach – assure them you're doing this to maintain your dignity and ensure that your wishes are carried out. Remind them as well, that if this situation should arise it would be a lot easier on them if your wishes were known in advance.

Should I talk about this with my doctor?

Yes! Bring it up at your next appointment or make a special appointment for this purpose. Talk honestly with your doctor about options that are right for you and the state of your disease.

How do I get started?

Your local hospital should have forms that are legal in your state, and they should have a social worker to assist you. A lawyer can also help you. There are many resources on the Internet. Just make sure that documents are legal in your state, as laws vary from state to state.

The charge for downloading or sending for such documents are generally affordable.

You might be wondering what happened with Dad. Well, after ten days in the ICU, he pulled through and lived for nearly two more years. He was well enough in that time to see grandchildren get married and graduate from college and high school – and he even went back to work part time. Also, in that time he made it clear to all of us exactly what he wanted should he ever be that sick again, and unable to speak for himself. Finally, when he had no fight left in him, he passed away quietly with no tubes, no machines, and no pain – with family at his side. Yes, it took a while for a proud man to talk about end-of-life care, but we're so glad he did.

Your Turn

Key points, or…if you don't remember anything else from this chapter, remember this:

- Everybody should have an advance directive.
- Providing an advance directive in writing assures that your wishes (not the wishes or assumptions of others) will be carried out if you are ever unable to speak for yourself.
- You should talk with your doctor about end-of-life issues.
- Completing a legal advance directive can be easy and inexpensive.

Ask yourself this:

- Do I have the two parts of an Advance Directive: Durable power of Attorney for Health Care and a Living Will?
- Do I know where it is?

- Do my advocates have copies?
- If I already have one, does it need to be updated?

This week:

- If you don't have an advance directive, talk with your loved ones about it.
- If you do have an advance directive, be proud that you have that out of the way and do something fun that has to do with living – not dying!

October – Week 2

Depression

"Never despair."

~ Horace

I'm fighting for every breath here, doc. I can't do anything I used to. I was a strong guy – a firefighter for goodness sake. Now I can barely carry my own garden hose! I can't sleep, I can't concentrate, I don't feel like doing anything anymore." Jerry sat across from Dr. Rogers and leaned forward with his elbows on his knees. He looked down and sighed. "I don't know, doc. This COPD thing has really knocked me down."

Jerry is experiencing a few of the many signs of clinical depression – and he's not alone. Depression is common in people with COPD. And why shouldn't it be? After all, it's like any other chronic disease, right? Well, maybe not. Experts are learning more about depression in people with COPD, and they're finding that there may be an even closer connection than we thought.

To start, let's take a quick look at COPD and how it can affect your emotional well-being. Left untreated, COPD can be a wasting disease. You begin to do less and less, becoming increasingly weak until you're unable to do much of anything at all. This can lead to diminished independence prompting feelings of anger, frustration, isolation, and loss of control. Once you're on this downward spiral, depression may not be far behind.

How do you know if you could be depressed?

What are the symptoms of depression?

- Loss of interest in favorite activities
- Always tired
- Frequent sadness
- Irritability
- Significant weight change
- Wishing to be left alone
- Hopelessness
- Trouble sleeping
- Lack of appetite
- Thoughts of death or suicide
- Feeling worthless or guilty
- Difficulty concentrating

If you feel this way, or are even beginning to feel this way, you may be heading for depression. If any of these symptoms start to creep up on you, take action.

What should you do?

- Tell your doctor if you have any of these symptoms.
- Ask him or her about anti-depressant medication and if this might be right for you.
- Ask your doctor if you should talk with a counselor or other mental health specialist. It is not a sign of weakness to talk with somebody about issues that affect your happiness and well-being. Really.
- Ask your doctor to refer you to pulmonary rehabilitation (see chapter January – Week 5). There you will learn how

to exercise safely and effectively even if you're very short of breath. This will help you build up your strength and use your oxygen more efficiently. The more fit you are, the more confidence you have, and the more your outlook improves. At pulmonary rehab you'll learn tips for staying healthy – and you'll meet others who understand what it's like to live each day with COPD.

- Talk with an understanding friend or clergy. Sometimes just sitting down and talking about what you're going through can make your problems easier to deal with.
- Give yourself a change of scene by taking a walk or drive. Just getting out of the house can help you feel much better. Seeing something new helps take your mind off yourself. If possible, make it a routine to get out of the house at least three times a week.
- Join a group – a local breathing support or one online, a harmonica group (see chapter September – Week 1) or one based on a hobby, like a book club, stamp collecting, quilting, something that makes you feel good. The wider you can make your circle of acquaintances, the better.
- Educate your family. As well intentioned as your loved ones may be, they often have no idea what it's like to live with COPD.
- Help others by volunteering. Even with shortness of breath, there are things you can do to make your community a better place. Check with your local hospital, school, house of worship, or library, and ask what you can do.

So, what did Dr. Rogers say? "Jerry, it sounds like you're depressed. I think we can help you with that."

"Oh, I don't know…maybe I'm just getting old."

"This happens to a lot of folks. I'm going to send you over to see

Lynda, the respiratory therapist at pulmonary rehab. She can tell you about the program. I think you could also benefit from talking with somebody about this."

"Now, wait a minute, doc…I'm not going to a shrink. I'll just give myself a kick and I'll be fine."

Dr. Rogers smiled. "Okay, no 'shrink,' for now. How about your pastor? I'll bet he'd be happy to take a few minutes to sit down and talk with you."

"Well, he's always asking me to stop in for coffee…"

"Good. Give him a call. Today. And one more thing – I'm giving you a prescription for an anti-depressant."

"Hold on now…I've never been one to…"

"Just give it a try, and if you don't think it's working, let me know. But I really think it'll help." He paused. "Okay, Jerry, are you all set? Anything else you want to ask me?"

"Nope, I think that's it, doc. Thanks."

Depression is common in people with COPD. But it's nothing to be ashamed of! Watch for the signs of depression, recognize them, accept them for what they are, talk to your doctor, and then follow through with the help that's available. Beware of that nasty monster – depression. He'll sneak up on you if you let him. But now that you know who he is, and what to do, you can fight him off – and get on with living.

Your Turn

Key points, or…if you don't remember anything else from this chapter, remember this:

- Depression is common in people with COPD.
- Being depressed does not mean you are weak-minded.

- Depression can be treated effectively in a variety of ways.
- It's important to watch for signs of depression and know that although well-controlled at one time, it may appear again.

Ask yourself this:

Do I have any symptoms of depression?

This week:

If you have symptoms of depression, make an appointment with your doctor to talk about it.

October – Week 3

Additional Therapies for COPD: Massage, Yoga, Tai chi, and Qigong

"When you're through changing, you're through."

~ Bruce Barton

When learning about living well with COPD, of course we should focus on the basics of good lung health, such as medications, nutrition, breathing techniques, exercise, etc. It's also important – essential, in fact – to pay close attention to emotional issues, such as anxiety, denial, and relationships, to name a few. But in this chapter, we're going to talk about some other forms of therapy that can add to good lung health and help you stay well with COPD. These are activities you might never have thought could have a positive effect on your breathing: yoga, tai chi, qigong, and massage.

Elsewhere in this book you'll find references to yoga and tai chi. In chapter July – Week 3: Relaxation, Dr. Sharma provides a step-by-step routine for relaxation and breathing related to yoga techniques. In chapter April – Week 4: Coping with Stress, Jo-Von Tucker talks briefly about the benefits of tai chi. Understand that things like yoga, tai chi, qigong, and massage are not meant to replace the treatment program prescribed by your doctor, but to enhance it. Always consult your doctor before starting any new therapy. Ask around and talk with people who have had the particular treatment you're considering.

Here is one lady's experience with massage and how it affected her life with very severe COPD. I know you'll find it interesting – and inspiring.

A classmate of mine in pulmonary rehab mentioned one day that she was getting massage for pain issues. She said she felt so much better and that she felt she could breathe better. And I could see that she did. She recommended I consider massage for myself and gave me the number of her massage therapist. So, skeptical as I was, I trusted my rehab friend and made an appointment with Terri.

I have to tell you…I'm not one of those women who go in for "spa days" and what I consider primping sorts of things. That's what I always thought massage was – like manicures and pedicures. Activities that are okay to do, I thought, but a waste of good money. I mean, I would rather buy a pair of shoes, or something for my grandson, or go out to lunch with a friend – anything but "waste" the money on myself!

Another reason I was hesitant to have a massage was my own vanity. I've lost so much weight and as you may know, the skin just doesn't shrink as we age! People think of me as being tiny. I'm 5'2" and weigh 97 pounds. One girl joked at pulmonary rehab that she was born larger than I am now! Others say I am so thin I might break! This is just my body, so I am not really aware of what they're referring to. On the other hand, I don't think others can picture me as I see myself – with saggy skin from severe weight loss, wrinkles and scars left by surgeries, and all of that. I used to be pretty strong – muscular to a point – well-toned and proud of how I looked in a bikini! No way, now!

But when the day came, I found the courage to go ahead and keep my appointment. I learned that my massage therapist has a nursing background and I think it is one reason she is so effective for someone with severe COPD like mine (I am down to around 19-20%

FEV$_1$). I was relieved, also, to find out that in massage, the therapist only uncovers whatever part of your body she is working on and never sees me completely undressed! If I had known that I might have gone sooner!

You might be concerned that during massage you must lie down on a flat surface. Some people with COPD can't lie flat and need to have their head raised. If this is the case, you can ask your massage therapist if he or she can work around that. I cannot go from moving around a lot, being winded, and then just lying down flat. But I can do it, if I do it in stages. Another of my concerns was about the cost. Just how much was this luxury going to set me back? Well, if I were still smoking it would be a little more than a carton of cigs.

I've now gone four weeks in a row, and even my husband is impressed with how much better I'm doing. At the first session, I talked my way through it – telling Terri about all my pain and what had caused it (surgeries and other injuries). The second time she had to wake me up. I gave in to relaxing to the feel of her hands and the sound of peaceful music. The last two sessions have been a combination.

Undeniably, I am breathing better and so much more relaxed. The tension she has been able to release from my muscles is amazing. My body was so tightened up it's surprising I was able to breathe at all!

I would highly recommend considering massage therapy to anyone, whether you're a man or a woman, with tension build-up, breathing issues, pain issues, or just in need of a "self-preservation" experience. I can state that for me, it was, and will continue to be, well worth the expense!

If you think massage might help you, ask your doctor if it would be safe for you to try. Ask others with COPD if they have experience with this and if they have someone they like. As always, when you have a chronic medical condition, be sure you're working with people who have:

- Accreditation and experience.
- A willingness to provide references.
- Experience working specifically on people with COPD.

Added Insight

Debbie's story – Tai chi and Qigong

After more than forty-five years of smoking, I quit once again, but this time it was for good. I needed something to help me cope. I wanted to replace smoking with something healthy. The goal was to quit smoking and work on my health.

Two years prior to this I had been diagnosed with COPD by my primary care physician. I had not yet seen a pulmonologist and knew nothing about pulmonary rehab. I was on my own to figure something out. I knew I needed to move, and I knew I needed something to help me cope with quitting smoking. Full blown exercise was not even on my radar – definitely not capable. I was just trying to not smoke and not fade away.

Qigong got me moving again, very slowly, but it was my first step and we all need to take that first step. For people with advanced COPD, that first step is a very big deal. Tai chi is rooted in the qigong tradition, but they are not the same. Tai chi is an ancient form of selfdefense and more physical, while qigong is an ancient form of selfhealing that involves movement with mindful meditation. Qigong is about easy, gentle movements without the intimidation of exercise. It's about mindfulness of being in motion while managing your breathing. It's awareness of your breathing without the fear. That is the biggest challenge with COPD – how to breathe and move without being afraid of getting breathless.

In terms of exercise I have come a long way and qigong is still fundamental to my self-help treatment. These days my exercise program addresses the cardio and the strength elements while qigong addresses my breathing. I practice qigong energy breathing at the gym when I get very short of breath and need to settle my breathing down. In that situation I do a type of qigong breathing that is basically pursedlips breathing; in a sense it is mindful pursed-lips breathing. I will do some tai chi qigong breathing briefly before I start an exercise that is difficult and tends to make me have lower oxygen saturations.

I practice a little qigong every morning before using my inhalers. It forces me to slow down, relax, and pay attention to what I am doing. By performing deep breathing exercises, I am able to take a deeper breath and hold it longer. I feel that I can use my inhalers more effectively.

Several times a week I do either one or two qigong practices. Baduanjin, or the Eight Pieces of the Silken Brocades, is a challenging practice, taking about twenty minutes to complete. I cannot do some parts of it, so I have adapted. If anyone thinks qigong is not exercise, I challenge them to do the full Eight Brocades and then tell me how their legs feel. Some days I want something easier, something to help me de-stress. The Xi Sui Jing known as the Bone Marrow Cleanse is perfect for that. It is more of a moving mediation.

It's all about breathing – mindful, deep breathing combined with gentle but purposeful movement. Qigong helps me stay in tune with my breathing – in a positive way.

Your Turn

Key points, or...if you don't remember anything else from this chapter, remember this:

- Keep your mind open to therapies that might enhance your existing COPD treatment program.
- Always consult your doctor before starting additional therapy.
- Check credentials and references of anybody who will be

coaching you on movement or performing body contact therapy.

Ask yourself this:

Could yoga, tai chi, qigong, or massage help me?

This week:

Ask a respiratory healthcare professional or peer if they would recommend this type of therapy.

October – Week 4
Losing Someone with COPD

"Life is a great sunrise. I do not see why death
should not be an even greater one."

~ Vladimir Nobokov

JVT

Sadly, we recently lost two of our COPD support group members. They passed away on the same day.

Elizabeth was such a gentle lady, and enthusiastic about joining our group and coming to meetings. Jack was just irrepressible – so full of life, and with such a zest for living! Jack, I believe, never met a stranger. He could – and did – converse with anyone who showed the least interest in talking with him. He took up many of the causes that were offered specifically for supplemental oxygen users and came away with many friends each time. He just had a special delight in his eyes...mischievous, yes...harmful to others, never!

Losing Jack has made me think about the valiant fight he put forth as he battled COPD. In recent months his health took a nosedive, and he struggled mightily to regain his strength and stamina. He never did.

But more than that, Jack's life was open, loving, accepting, and totally nonjudgmental. We can all learn from that. And we can all strive to embrace the positive aspects of our lives now, even with COPD. Just as Jack did.

Okay, I know it's no fun living with this disease. But we still have our vision, allowing us to see the beautiful things – and people – around us. We still have our hearts, although they may be a little rusty from the strain of pumping against impaired lung function, but allow us feelings of love and affection, or so the fable of the heart goes.

Some of us still have our hearing, which results in receiving pleasant sounds and wonderful music, of soft voices and the laughter of babies. We can listen when friends and family talk to us, and really hear the meaning behind the words.

We still have our brains, mostly intact, which let us remember the good times and the great people we've known, some who came directly from our involvement with our breathing support group.

We still have a lot to be thankful for, and there are many more good aspects of life to come. Sometimes it takes the loss of a friend to make us realize that, in spite of COPD, we can enjoy a really good life.

We can still laugh, and yes, sometimes we cry. We may not be able to run anymore, but we can walk. Most of all, we must remember that we should never, ever take for granted the life we live.

Take a page from Jack's book. Live your life with joy in your heart, and don't be afraid to share it with others.

Losing Friends in Pulmonary Rehab *JMM*

In memory of "The Three Amigos," Arnie, Les, and Merle.

Probably the hardest aspect of my job as a respiratory therapist in pulmonary rehab was when a patient in our program died. The participants in our groups became friends, even like family. When a member of our group passed away, others in the class, as well as our staff, couldn't help but be affected.

So, what to do? How to cope when you know you all have the same, or similar, incurable, progressive disease? Even if the person who died didn't pass away as a direct result of his or her COPD, their passing reminds us of our own mortality. Sometimes classmates wondered aloud, "Am I next?"

As we processed the loss, we as a pulmonary rehab program had our own special ways to grieve, remember, and honor the memory of our classmates. Maybe the classmate we lost was quiet and reserved. Maybe he or she was the class clown or perhaps the nurturer, the den mother or father figure. No matter what, we were thankful for the way in which they contributed to our group. I hope you have special observances you do that hold meaning for you.

Here are some things we did – call them customs, call them rituals, we called them honoring our friends. We called them comforting.

I was usually the first one to hear that a member of our class had died. In getting ready for that person's class to come in, I'd set up a picture in the sign-in area of our lost classmate, along with his or her obituary. This way, participants knew at the beginning of class what had happened. They then had a minimum of one hour together to share memories, or at the very least, not be alone.

A dear lady in one class would bring in a long-stemmed cut flower and place it on the chair where that person sat. We all, classmates and staff, signed a sympathy card to send to the family. If possible, some staff and classmates individually attended the wake, visitation, or funeral. It meant so much to the family to meet people who knew their loved one. Even though most family members had not met the people from pulmonary rehab, they felt they knew us because they'd heard their loved one talk about us often at home. If we couldn't attend services or visitation, we sometimes made a short phone call to a family member.

Some participants in our program had learned how to raise

monarch butterflies. It's a tradition to name a monarch when it is released – to give it the name of someone lost within the past year. Seeing a brand-new butterfly spread its wings and fly, while calling it by the name of your lost loved one, is a healing experience and an affirmation that life does go on.

Yes, our grief is deep when we lose a friend in our pulmonary rehab, local harmonica group, or online breathing support group. But, as a class, a group, peers, students, or friends, you can share your grief, your joy, even your tears. It doesn't make it any easier, but it can give you comfort. You and your peers may honor your lost friend, each in your own way. But together you honor them by being thankful they were a part of your experience, your journey with COPD.

Added Insight

A poem by Mary Elizabeth Frye

Do Not Stand at My Grave and Weep

Do not stand at my grave and weep
I am not there, I do not sleep
I am a thousand winds that blow
I am the diamond glint on snow
I am the sunlight on ripened grain
I am the gentle autumn rain
When you wake in the morning hush
I am the swift, uplifting rush
Of quiet birds in circling flight
I am the soft starlight at night
Do not stand at my grave and cry.
I am not there, I did not die!

Your Turn

Key points, or…if you don't remember anything else from this chapter, remember this:

- It's a fact of life that at some time or another we will lose friends and loved ones who have the same, or similar health issue.
- Spending time with others who knew that person can help. Even if you don't talk, it is good to be together.
- Participating in customs or rituals is comforting and helps us heal, even though we're still sad.

Ask yourself this:

Do I express appreciation, even if it's just a smile or friendly hello, to those I know who have serious health problems?

This week:

Take special notice of the positive qualities in those you know and love and tell them you appreciate them.

November – Week I

Isolation with COPD and Why We Need Emotional Support

"Individually, we are one drop. Together, we are an ocean."

~ Ryunosuke Satoro

Someone in the medical profession once said to me, "People with COPD are like old Indians...they tend to just fade away." What that person was referring to was the fact that many of us tend to disappear from the public eye, to stay at home where it is easier and more comfortable than venturing out. COPD itself isn't to blame for the isolation. We aren't contagious. But there are many considerations that lead to our decision to "stay in."

A serious lack of energy is one of the reasons we tend to stay at home. Getting ready to be seen by the outside world requires a great deal of effort. We need to shower, maybe shampoo, shave or apply makeup, and dress. These are not small tasks when each one may send us grasping for our puffers and gasping for breath.

Then there is the issue of awkwardness. We may be embarrassed when we're out in public because of sensitivity about our oxygen equipment, or because we may be seized with a spell of uncontrollable coughing. We might feel uncomfortable because we can only walk for short distances before exhaustion sets in, or perhaps because people stare at us. Maybe we simply don't feel well. It's difficult to get out and about on those bad days. All of these are reasons we can become mired in isolation.

Isolation is a killer for COPD patients. It may take us away far sooner than even a series of exacerbations. It is something we need to fight with all the energy we can muster, because the alternative is simply to give in to seclusion – and cause us to just fade away!

Granted, it takes a lot of effort for us to socialize. And no one around us will ever understand the price we pay to go to a movie or have lunch with friends. It will never occur to them the kind of effort it takes for us to get out to enjoy a birthday party. Nor should it. We need to realize that we are the ones who must be aware of the importance of getting on with our lives, and to do it with all the quality we can hold onto. We should not depend on others – even caregivers or mates – to provide us with entertainment and a reason to live.

As people with COPD, we don't have to be isolated. By being realistic about our abilities as well as our limitations, we can implement a plan that will provide us with plenty of reasons to get up each day. Here is a list of relatively easy-to-do activities, even for COPD'ers.

- Make a list of people you enjoy being with – people who are good for you – people who have a positive attitude and understand your COPD. Plan some activities or events that will allow you to spend time with them. Refer to your list often and remind yourself why you need to be with them.
- Plan your calendar, keeping in mind the activities that take the most effort. Space your outings so there is plenty of rest time in between.
- Keep things simple! If you are inviting folks over for lunch, plan a menu that will be easy, not one that requires huge amounts of effort. Choose a salad that can be prepared the day before. Select a dessert you can pick up from the local bakery. It's the company that counts, not the praise for being a great host.

Make a list of activities you really like to do. Is it reading, playing bridge, attending craft fairs, playing with your grandchildren, baking, solving puzzles, updating a scrapbook or family photo album, corresponding with faraway friends? How about going to the movies, lunch or dinner out, attending church or synagogue, or going for a scenic drive? These are things you can plan to enjoy with someone, breaking the isolation. The important thing is to do them! Don't just plan. Carry them out! Imagine how much better you will feel for the company, for the activity, for the experience. Your heart will be lighter, and so will the burden of your disease.

We can't forget how much it can help to go to support group meetings. Involvement in a COPD support group is a good place to start breaking a habit of isolation. The people you'll meet there share many of the same symptoms, concerns, and issues. It really does help to go to meetings – to listen, to talk, to learn, to exchange experiences, and to share feelings with those who truly understand how we feel.

Pulmonary rehab is another great way to get out and meet people who understand what we're going through. Even if you don't feel like going anywhere, if you're not sick that day, you should push yourself to get there. After we do, we're so glad we did!

Finally, avoiding isolation and getting out is a commitment to ourselves that we are working to feel better, or at least remain stable. It is a commitment we should be happy to make, for the results of our involvement far outweigh our effort. We'll feel so much better because of the company, the activity, the experience. Our hearts will be lighter and so will the burden of our disease.

Living with COPD is not a death sentence. It's a journey. And when you're walking a path you've never been on before, it sure does help to have some friends with a map.

Your Turn

Key points, or…if you don't remember anything else from this chapter, remember this:

- No matter if you have mild COPD, severe COPD, or something in between, try to avoid isolation as much as possible.
- You can still enjoy a social life, even if you are significantly limited by your COPD.
- Becoming involved in a breathing support group and/or pulmonary rehab is a good place to start and a great way to meet others.

Ask yourself this:

Do I regularly get out into public and socialize with others? If so, what do I do? If not, why not?

This week:

Do at least one of the following:

- Find your nearest breathing support group and make plans to go.
- Find your nearest pulmonary rehabilitation program, talk with the staff and ask if it would be appropriate for you to enroll. If so, call your doctor and ask for a referral.
- Call a friend or family member and set a date to do something you enjoy.

November – Week 2

Ten Tips to Enjoy the Holidays

"Don't let what you cannot do interfere with what you can do."

~ John Wooden

If you're healthy and free of chronic disease, the holidays can be stressful enough. But, if you have COPD you might be looking at the holidays with downright fear and dread, and be inclined to say, "It's such a hassle. I'm tempted to forget the whole thing and just stay home." But it really doesn't need to be that way!

Here are ten tips to help you enjoy the holidays, even if you have COPD. This is, by no means, a complete list – it's just a start to show you that with a little planning, you *can* get out, participate in holiday events and enjoy the season with family and friends.

1. **Scented candles** – If you're going to a party or gathering where you expect there might be scented candles, call ahead and gently ask your host if they wouldn't mind not lighting them that day, or at least until after you've left the party. Explain that the scent irritates your lungs and you won't be able to appreciate the party if the candles get in the way of your ability to breathe.

2. **Park close or get dropped off** – Don't find yourself walking farther than you're comfortably able to walk, especially in the

cold air. If you're riding with someone, ask if they can drop you off at the door. If you're doing the driving, call ahead to your host and ask if you can drive up to the door and someone at the party (perhaps a responsible teen driver) can serve as a valet. This is where having a cell phone comes in handy. In fact, everybody with COPD should have a fully charged cell phone when they venture away from home!

3. **Don't eat too much** – All those goodies are tempting, but overeating can expand your stomach to the point that it pushes up on your already compromised diaphragm. If you want to try everything, just take little bits and bites; don't gobble it all down at once but stretch it out over time.

4. **Give yourself time** – Rushing and hurrying is a huge problem for people with breathing problems who simply can't move fast. Allow for plenty of time to get ready so you'll arrive when you want, you'll look beautiful/handsome (whatever the case may be) and have breath to spare!

5. **Avoid nasty germs** – Stay away from small children who are coughing and sneezing. They can shake off a cold virus. You can't. At their age they don't know enough to cover their mouth and nose. Avoid shaking hands and kissing on the lips. The Hollywood "air kiss" or an elbow touch works just fine! When you've weathered the winter without an exacerbation, you'll be happy you did – or didn't!

6. **Cover up** – Wear a mask or scarf over your nose and mouth in cold air to keep your airways from having spasms, which can cause an uncontrollable cough and more shortness of breath.

7. **Delegate** – Shop for gifts online. If you can't, ask somebody to go shopping with you or to pick up a specific, easy-to-find gift when they're out doing their shopping. If the party is at your house, don't do all the work! Involve your guests and assign tasks. Children, and yes, even teens, are usually willing

to help. It will enrich their lives to learn about your physical limitations and it will make them feel proud to know they've helped out.

8. **Be a Santa** – Surprise somebody by doing something nice. Send a note to your neighbor or phone a friend with a brief and cheerful, "I'm just thinking about you and wanted to wish you a 'Merry Christmas' or 'Happy Holidays.'" Make cookies or a quick bread for your letter carrier. Don't underestimate the power of a small kindness or show of appreciation. Little things really do mean a lot!

9. **Enjoy the moments** – Live in the moment. If you're breathing well at the moment, smile, laugh, and enjoy the party! Don't spend your energy worrying about tomorrow. This very day – the time you're in right now – will never come along again. All of us are promised only today, nothing else.

10. **It's their problem** – Don't beat yourself up over what you might have done in the past to cause damage to your lungs. You're not the only person at that party who may have done something bad for their health. You're doing the very best you can right now to be healthy, and if somebody can't deal with that, it's their problem. If you use supplemental oxygen (and we say supplemental because *everybody* uses oxygen) think of it this way: Some people use bottled water, you just use bottled air!

Your Turn

Key points, or…if you don't remember anything else from this chapter, remember this:

- Plan ahead.
- Know your limits.

- Cherish the moment.
- Have fun!

Ask yourself this:

- What was a problem for me last year?
- Can any of these suggestions help make my holidays more enjoyable this year?

This week:

Think about an upcoming event and plan so that can be enjoyable for you.

November – Week 3

A Time of Thanksgiving

"Not what we say about our blessings, but how we use them, is the true measure of our thanksgiving."

~ W.T. Purkiser

In the United States we honor a tradition with our observance of Thanksgiving Day, a day of family and feasting, and expressing our thanks for all we have.

It seems to me that those of us with COPD may recognize our own special reasons to celebrate and give thanks. Our perspective, coming from that of being diagnosed with a chronic, progressive, so-far-incurable disease, may differ from others in our world. This is because it comes from the unique mindset of someone who must struggle each day to breathe well and survive to see tomorrow.

Let's count our blessings together. Yours may be different than mine, but I know we share many of the same reasons to give thanks. I picture a cornucopia, not with what I don't have, but with what I do. Here's what I see:

- I am grateful to have the strength it takes to get up and face each new day.
- I give thanks for each time I am able to avoid a lung infection.
- I am more appreciative than ever of the beauty that surrounds

me – in nature, in my life, in my heart.

- I am thankful for the support and understanding of my family and good friends.
- I am glad I have more good days than bad ones.
- I am pleased I can rely on my doctor and healthcare team in times of need.
- I am grateful for the friends I have made in our support group – people who truly understand how I feel.
- I am deliriously happy with the extra mobility that my portable oxygen system provides, and with the innovations in supplemental oxygen delivery systems.
- I am delighted to know that research is taking place to hopefully provide insight and help for all COPD'ers.
- I am grateful for the pleasure I derive from short walks by the ocean.
- I am happy I can occasionally dream that I am healthy again, freed in my dreams from the disability of COPD.
- If you are lucky enough to have a spouse who watches over you and helps you, you are glad for the ability to say, "Thank You!" to him or her.

Thanksgiving does not have to be marked on a calendar. It can be honored each day. It doesn't need to be accompanied by roast turkey and all the trimmings. It can be a quiet, solitary meal, or a simple acknowledgement of the importance of those individuals who affect our lives so deeply now. You know who they are, and so should they.

As pulmonary patients, our perspectives may be different, but our passions are as strongly felt as anyone else's. And I suspect that the gratitude we feel for the continuation of the good things in our lives may be even more heartfelt, because we are constantly at risk of losing them.

Each of us occasionally gives in to brief bouts of grieving for the things we can no longer do or have. However, as the changes in our lifestyles have taken place, so, too, have new opportunities found their way to us. The new doors that have opened are the ones we must focus on now. They are the promise of good times to come, of cherished memories – and new beginnings.

Those newly discovered opportunities are huge reasons themselves, for our gratitude. *Anticipation, excitement, joy, and a sense of accomplishment* – all are by-products of taking on new responsibilities and learning about new pleasures. All can bring renewal and rediscovery to each of us. I am so grateful to be aware of them in my life.

When I face each day as a precious gift, I feel grateful. The gift of a new day is the best one we can expect to receive. Think about it...with the dawn of each new day it's like getting God's okay to have another go at it. So, let's take it, do our best, and just say, "Thank you."

Added Insight

John Smith's thoughts on being thankful

It was the Tuesday before Thanksgiving. The members of the eleven o'clock pulmonary rehabilitation phase three maintenance class sat together, waiting for class to start. John Smith slowly stood, white folded paper in hand, and shared the following with the group – his thoughts on Thanksgiving.

I was reminded one recent Sunday morning that I should try to be thankful for adversity and challenges in my life. I have a pulmonary problem. How can I possibly be *thankful* for this breathing challenge?

I thought of my pulmonary rehab class. The need for discipline and exercise in breathing brought me into this class and in contact with its leaders and classmates. It is these people who give to me my reason for thanksgiving. Because of them my life is fuller, more enriched. But how is this possible? I'll tell you.

I had some concern about my grandson. Jane, a respiratory

therapist, has teenagers herself. She assured me not to be discouraged. "It will all work out alright," she said. Without her assurance, worry would have eaten away at me. I am thankful for Jane. I am thankful for acceptance and assurance.

Lynda, a nurse, is concerned about areas of my health other than pulmonary. She shows concern about my heart and fluid balance, and sometimes insists I contact my internist. I am thankful for Lynda. I am thankful for vigilant healthcare professionals.

Ruth always asks, "How are you feeling today, John?" If she didn't ask, I wouldn't know that someone really cares. I am thankful for Ruth. I am thankful for sincere concern.

Can my adversity be met and overcome? I know it can! Bud has shown this to me by his perseverance through a lung transplant. It may take months or years, but improvement is possible. I am thankful for Bud. I am thankful for witnessing the miracle of organ donation and perseverance in the face of overwhelming odds.

Dave has a caustic wit that cheers me up. Without him I might not know that merriness can be so close at hand. With Dave in the class, I can laugh. I am thankful for Dave. I am thankful for laughter.

Bernie and Shirley remind me that God is still on the throne. I need to visit with them while exercising. They reassure me in a spiritual way. If I did not have this breathing problem I would not be in rehab and would miss out on the conversations we have. Bernie and Shirley are a beautiful couple. I am thankful for them. I am thankful for lasting faith.

Glenn and I have mutual friends. He keeps me posted on their whereabouts. Without his sharing in rehab, who would keep me in touch? I am thankful for Glenn. I am thankful for connectedness.

One of my rehab classmates is a man from Cambodia. Om reminds me that life reaches past my background and around the world. Although he understands little English, Om always has a bright and cheerful smile for me. My life would be less without him. I am thankful for Om. I am thankful for smiles.

Mitzi shares with me her love and knowledge of classical music. She also communicates her concern about world events. Mitzi is a serious conversationalist. She makes me think. I am thankful for Mitzi. I am thankful for a new friend with sharp intellect.

For all the others in the class who inspire me with their determination, and for the staff members who help me, I am thankful. So now, because of my breathing problem, my life has become enriched. I have found joy and contentment in the midst of adversity. I am thankful for my pulmonary struggle. And I am thankful for the richness it brings.

Your Turn

Key points, or…if you don't remember anything else from this chapter, remember this:

- It's good for us to be thankful for whatever we have.
- We can find many things to be thankful for if we just take the time to notice them.
- Having COPD may take some things away, but it can also give us new opportunities.

Ask yourself this:

Because I have COPD, what good things are in my life now that I didn't have before?

This week:

Find something to be thankful for each day this week and write it down in the chart on the next page. On the seventh day look back on your list and see all those good things.

Find something to be thankful for each day this week, and write it down. On the seventh day look back on your list and see all those good things.

SUNDAY	Today I am thankful for _____ _____ _____
MONDAY	Today I am thankful for _____ _____ _____
TUESDAY	Today I am thankful for _____ _____ _____
WEDNESDAY	Today I am thankful for _____ _____ _____
THURSDAY	Today I am thankful for _____ _____ _____
FRIDAY	Today I am thankful for _____ _____ _____
SATURDAY	Today I am thankful for _____ _____ _____

November – Week 4

Dear Family and Friends, In a Perfect World...

"Learn what you are, and be such."

~ Pindar

Dear Family and Friends,

Our lives may never be quite the same, A.D. (after diagnosis). In a perfect world, I wouldn't have COPD. But we can all try to seek more joy, derive more pleasure, from what we are fortunate enough to have – one another. Let's make the most of our time.

In a perfect world, you wouldn't have to wonder how I was feeling, and wonder what you might be able to do to help me. You wouldn't find yourself on the receiving end of my emotions related to the depression to which I am prone. Nor would you have to puzzle over the fact that I seem to have good days, and then unexplainably, so many bad days.

You must be terribly disturbed by my shortness of breath, and by the fatigue that nibbles at me all day, every day. And I can guess that you are as upset and embarrassed as I am by the fits of coughing that sometimes seize me, especially out in public.

You know that the compromises to my lifestyle are upsetting. It's hard for me to ask for help when I find that I can no longer do something on my own. It hurts my pride, and I can see in your eyes that it hurts you, too.

But this isn't a perfect world, is it? I do have this disease, and so far, there is no cure. I must learn to cope with it. We all must. So, even though the world is less than perfect, particularly since being diagnosed with COPD, these issues do exist.

I want to find a way to help you as you try to help me. That's why I'm writing this letter to you now. Sometimes it's just easier to write things down than it is to say them out loud – especially things that cause this big lump in my throat, even as I write.

You are my loved and cherished family. And it seems to me that family members are often hit as hard with the realities of COPD as the patient. Maybe even harder. It pains me to see you struggle with solutions as we fight the battle of this disease together. I know you want to help.

Our lives inexplicably intertwined by the fact that I have this disease. But I have learned COPD is not a death sentence, nor does it have to be the end of our quality of life. The better I become at managing my own disease, the more effective and happier our time together will be. Maybe if we establish some ground rules, we can get through the rough patches and adapt more easily and with less stress on us all.

Here is my fantasy of what our nearly perfect world could be – despite COPD – within my list of seven suggestions:

1. It is important for me to remain as independent as possible to preserve my self-esteem. Try not to rush over to help me before you know whether or not I can accomplish a task on my own. I really want to try; not only to spare you, but also to help me with my independence and self-esteem, both of which will erode significantly with everything I learn I can't do.

There is a fine line that you, my dear ones, must walk in balancing between coming to my aid, or just taking over for me (which can be interpreted as enabling me to become a cripple). This is important for many reasons; here are just two: The need to keep my body and muscles as conditioned and toned as possible, and the need I have to feel useful again – to help guard against a loss of self-esteem.

2. Try to not judge me if I'm having a bad day. It is possible that a lung infection could be brewing. In fact, you may be aware of it sooner than I am myself. You know the signs: increased shortness of breath and coughing up discolored sputum, perhaps fever, but maybe not, and less energy for the simple chores of daily living.

Some of the folks in my lung support group have expressed their frustration when their family leaps to the conclusion that we are hypochondriacs who complain a lot about feeling bad. This just isn't so; we aren't constant complainers. COPD'ers are a pretty brave lot. Most of us who have COPD do not want our loved ones to see us as "sickly" or making excuses. As a result, however, many of us hedge about the problems we are experiencing.

3. Please help me by overseeing that I am complying with the treatment plan my doctor has prescribed. I don't expect you to be a nurse, but I appreciate it if you gently remind me to take my afternoon puffs on my inhalers or check to see if I remembered to take my evening pills. Help me be a compliant patient by assisting with my oxygen equipment when we go out. It's good to know I have a portable filled with enough supplemental oxygen to get me comfortably through our schedule.

It's also good to have help getting in and out of the car, and especially helpful to have an arm to lean on going up stairs, if I need it. The more comfortable we all are with the oxygen and equipment, the sooner it will be accepted and not questioned by the general public.

4. Help me stay socialized. Do not let me become isolated from friends and other family members. We COPD folks do tend to stay at home rather than digging down deep for the energy to get up and out! You can encourage me to go with you to lunch, or even to the market. You can inspire me to go to a movie or to have guests in for a game of cards. Your encouragement makes the difference for me – desiring to see people, and for people to see me!

5. In this nearly perfect world, we need to have and show respect for one another. I promise I won't talk about you as if you aren't in the room, if you'll do the same for me. My feelings are worn very close to the surface; I can hear perfectly well what you've said to someone about how fast the disease is progressing, or about how futile our efforts to fight it may seem. You and I can certainly discuss these issues between ourselves and keep them within the family circle.

6. Encourage me (but please don't nag me) about getting my exercises in each day. Some days it is just so hard to commit to even ten minutes of active exercises. If I'm too sick to do them myself, try to help me with just some stretching exercises like yoga or tai chi. These gentle movements help to keep my body conditioned even when I'm suffering from an exacerbation. And they aren't that taxing of my strength or

energy. You, of course, no matter how hard you try, cannot fully understand how I am feeling because you don't have COPD. But your encouragement brings me added strength; your emotional support brings me peace from the trauma of being sick.

7. Nutrition is an important part of helping my body with its special needs. You can help by making sure I'm eating right. A diet high in protein will help build up my immune system and body strength. We can plan the week's menus together. I pledge to try and tell you what items seem to taste best to me.

That's it...I'll stop with lucky number seven. I don't wish to make our lives more difficult with suggestions and rules. I simply want to express myself on the subject of how you can help me. I don't want to sound as though I am whining or complaining. I am reaching out with all the love in my heart for the help I know you want to provide. And if you have your own list of suggestions, please share them with me.

It is true that our lives may never be quite the same. But we can work together to preserve and enhance what we are fortunate enough to have – one another. Help me continue to fight on, to be stable, to endure what I will not let bring me down. Let's make the most of our time.

From my heart to yours,
Your Person with COPD

Your Turn

Key points, or…if you don't remember anything else from this chapter, remember this:

- Your family members want to help you in the best way possible. Sometimes they just don't know how.
- Open communication with your family and friends will help you all to understand how to cope with COPD.

Ask yourself this:

Have I told my loved ones what I need from them and what I don't need?

This week:

If this letter explains the way you feel, show it to your family and/or friends. If you feel differently, think about writing your own letter.

December – Week I
War or Peace?

"Acceptance doesn't mean you're giving up, or giving in. It means, simply, that you're smart enough to know what's going on. Then you can do what you need to do to live your life as well as you can."

~ Paige Sheridan

No matter what spiritual belief you may, or may not have, the holiday season should be a time of peace and well-being. The ideal would be to enjoy peace with our family, our friends, and our fellow man. But is it possible to make peace with a raging chronic disease that at times seems to spiral out of control, beyond our reach, with as little as a cough or sneeze? And how to have peace with ourselves if some choices we may have made in the past have led in part, to our COPD?

Have you ever noticed that some people seem to cope, emotionally, with COPD much better than others? Why is that? Possibly because they've found a way to stop being angry with themselves, making their way past the rage that often comes as a part of living with COPD.

Perhaps they have learned, also, to avoid – or at least work through – the occasional bouts of depression that commonly come with COPD. They have accepted the role of exercise as a vital part of their routine and most of them follow the treatment plan of their pulmonary doctor, actively involved in the management of their

COPD. They are educated about their disease. They are knowledge-able about their boundaries – when to push them, when to conserve precious energy, and how to make choices that will preserve their quality of life – even with the physical restrictions with which they are presented.

What about smoking? Those of us who were smokers, or still may be, often have an ongoing struggle with quitting – or staying quit. It can help to avoid fighting mode by simply accepting the fact that we are former smokers and always will be. The best we can do is to take one day at a time with the goal to not smoke today.

It isn't easy to make peace with COPD. It's a constant presence in the lives of us who live with it. It has a profound impact on our emotional health, self-image, relationships, work habits, aspirations, and overall outlook on life. And our struggle with it can cause us to feel like we've lost control of not only our breathing, but our lives.

It's interesting that the language of disease is a language of combat. We battle cancer, fight infections, overcome paralysis, conquer our fears. Disease is an enemy to be fought, and chronic disease is an enemy that is ever present, threatening us with chaos at any time. The war imagery obligates us to resist. On the other hand, looking at ourselves as "victims" of disease indicates that we are passive, when, in fact, chronic disease demands an active response.

What should we do? Should we fight the illness to the death, accepting it as our own normal state of being, or live in constant fear of being at the mercy of the next cough or sneeze? As COPD patients, we are neither perfectly healthy nor hopelessly ill. Choice is our right – but balance should be our goal.

Here is a list of scenarios, each with two extreme choices and a broad spectrum of responses. Neither of these extremes is healthy and they, each in their own way, put us at war with COPD. Where are you?

- You can tough it out, ignoring symptoms at the risk of getting worse – or you can check out every little quirk, at the risk of hypochondria.
- You can shop for miracle cures at the risk of harming yourself – or you can blindly trust one doctor's judgment at the risk of selecting unwisely.
- You can talk about it often at the risk of self-pity – or you can keep your disease secret at the risk of deception.
- You can hold fast to your independence at the risk of isolation and pushing yourself too far – or you can constantly ask friends for help at the risk of becoming a burden.
- You can insist that your family treat you as normal and healthy at the risk of denying them to be concerned about you – or you can let them coddle you at the risk of becoming overly dependent and child-like.
- You can strain your body to its limits at the risk of harming yourself – or you can play it too safe at the risk of becoming an invalid.
- You can look upon each good day as if you've "beaten the system" at the risk of smugness – or you can live in terror of degeneration and death at the risk of being emotionally paralyzed.
- You can insist on controlling every single aspect of your life at the risk of frustration – or you can "go with the flow" at the risk of passivity and victimization.
- You can be angry about your fate at the risk of bitterness – or you can focus only on your blessings at the risk of self-delusion.

War or Peace? The choices we make each day determine how we live with COPD. It isn't easy, but we can live in peace with COPD by having the grace of acceptance, and the determination to seek improvement. No doubt there will be days in which we won't make the right choices, but we'll learn from our mistakes. And we will keep on trying and also learn from others. With good choices, we'll have the peace that comes with doing the best we can under all circumstances. Our own balanced and centered life will get us through the rough times, and will define who we are, with or without COPD.

Added Insight

Quitting Smoking – Letters of support from Betty, Linda, Kay, Arlene, and John

Not all COPD is caused by cigarette smoking, * but let's face it – most of it, about 85% is. If you smoked cigarettes (or are still a smoker) and have COPD, you may feel guilty or ashamed for "bringing this on yourself."

So, how do you make peace with the thought of having an incurable, progressive disease that could have been prevented? First, know you're not the only person who ever smoked and ended up with COPD. There are millions like you. Next, know that you can find support from those who have been there – support in quit-smoking classes, breathing support groups, and pulmonary rehabilitation. The people there are ready to help you. Ask your doctor about recommending a quit method that may work for you. Choose a quit date that's meaningful to you and/ or a loved one: a birthday, anniversary, graduation, etc., with hopes for celebrating many more to come! Whatever you do, just start. Take one step at a time, and if you fall down, just get up and keep on trying.

Here are some letters of support from former smokers who were heavily addicted to nicotine. They did it. I hope you can, too.

Dear Betty,

I can relate. I was afraid to give up cigarettes, as they were my best friends. I thought an hour without one seemed impossible, so I began by doing without one for only five minutes at a time. I had a desire to smoke, but it went away whether I smoked or not. That's how I

got through it. If it were easy, everyone would quit. It was the hardest thing I ever did, but that keeps some of the guilt in check. Remember, you will go though many emotions and should feel free to express them. Don't keep your fears to yourself. Good luck."
Linda

Hi Kay!

Just wanted to let you know that the craving does lessen. The more time that goes by, the less the urge. For me, it was hard to get past that hand-mouth thing. So, I stuffed my mouth with hard candy and food; not the best way...just substituting one addiction for another. When I quit, I didn't know that the car would start without a cigarette, or that I could talk on the phone without one. Tea, alone? Without a butt? Impossible! But that passed.

For a long time after I quit, I had the smoking dream...the one where I would light up and wake up in a panic, breaking out into a cold sweat. It was before my COPD diagnosis...during my long denial period, and yet...even then, I knew that one more butt would kill me because there was no such thing as only 'one.'

Today, I rarely get the urge except after I put the Thanksgiving turkey in the oven...in years past that was the time I would sit for a few minutes, feet up, and light up...a short break before beginning the rest of the cooking. For the last three years, we've visited a dear friend for that holiday...no more urges for that day!

Seriously, it really does pass...it's just hard to see when recovery is so new...so take it one day at a time...it's the only way to survive it!
Arlene

I quit smoking three times before the success would last. The first time I threw my cigarettes out the car window. I just threw them out. And I went through all the cravings for about six months. The second time I took a Smoke Stoppers class through work. The third time, I

went out and bought a pound of candy – you know, all the mixed candies you buy in bulk. Every time I craved a cigarette, I'd have a piece of candy. I never really liked sweets. About halfway through the second pound, I just quit. That was it. I quit for good.
John

Finally, here is a letter to all the new quitters in a COPD online support group. The cheerleader is Janie in Sacramento, California.

Hello Everyone,
It's been a week now since you had that last cigarette. And this isn't the letter I had prepared for the first anniversary week for new non-smokers. The original was pretty typical jargon; you know, the 'atta girl' and 'atta boy' routine.
Then yesterday I heard the results of a Pulmonary Function test from one of my best friends who recently celebrated her 60th birthday. Due primarily to not being able to stop smoking, her lung function had dropped 10% in the past two and a half years. She had felt so guilty about smoking that she canceled checkups with her pulmonary doctor until she stopped three months ago.
It made me wonder how highly intelligent men and women could fall prey to a tobacco leaf that only an insect would eat. It made me wonder how easy it is for us to say, 'I'll think about that tomorrow' or 'I'll stop as a New Year's resolution next year.' It made me wonder why we ignored the warning signs. It made me wonder about a lot of things we would rather not confront.
For all of you out there who are 'hanging in there,' you should be very proud of what you are doing for yourselves and for your families. If you temporarily fail, dust yourself off and get back up again. But don't stop trying!
Playing solitaire in your bathrobe 24/7 is better than O_2 24/7. Eating carrot sticks, lemon drops, jellybeans, or carrying water

everywhere is better than having a cigarette. I once knew a CEO who ate toothpicks after he gave up smoking. He nibbled them and then spit out the little pieces of wood during board meetings. Disgusting to eat wood? And okay to ingest tobacco smoke? Well, you decide.

Just don't give up! We are cheering for all of you…those of you who were brave enough to come out and admit to everyone that you were trying to quit, and those of you who are quietly trying to stop in your own way. We are here to help you to find a better life than tobacco can give you…we're listening!
Janie in Sacramento

*Other causes of smoking are hazardous work environments, repeated lung infections early in life, and genetically inherited Alpha-1 Antitrypsin Deficiency.

Your Turn

Key points, or…if you don't remember anything else from this chapter, remember this:

- It is normal, and human, to feel as if you're at war with your COPD.
- You can learn how to keep a balance in order to be in control of your disease, and your life.

Ask yourself this:

Where am I on the spectrum of responses to my life with COPD?

This week:

Try to avoid extremes. Have balance in the choices you make to live in peace with COPD.

December – Week 2

Party Time! Nine Tips to Help You Save Energy and Breathe Better this Holiday Season

"Nothing is particularly hard if you divide it into small jobs."

~ Henry Ford

The holidays are upon us, and if you're anything like me, you're wondering how you're going to keep up with everything and still have time to enjoy this merry season. If you're living with COPD you might be thinking, "I barely have enough energy, and enough breath, as it is. With all there is to do, how can I possibly get through the holidays?"

Below are some tips to help you conserve that precious energy – and breath – so you can have a joyful holiday season. In chapter November – Week 2 we talked about some general holiday issues to consider. Here, we're going to talk specifically about **saving your energy** to make holiday tasks easier.

1. **Prioritize –** Which events do you really want to attend, and which ones are actually more an obligation to make someone else happy? Do what means the most to *you* and politely tell the other hosts that you have only so much breath to go around. Offer to do something fun with them after the first of

the year when life is not so hectic.

2. **Position yourself** – If you're at a family gathering and you want to help but don't have a lot of energy or endurance, ask if there is something you can do while sitting down. Maybe you can arrange a veggie or deli platter, fold napkins, or wrap gifts. If you have trouble standing for an extended period of time, don't volunteer to do the dishes. Rather, you might sit at the table and dry them. Guys…this goes for you, too!

3. **Plan ahead** – Being in a hurry is one of the biggest breath-robbers for people with COPD! Give yourself plenty of time to get ready, gather your goodies, and arrive at your destination with breath to spare.

4. **Place yourself** – Don't sit near triggers such as cooking fumes, steamy pots, scented candles, or stuffy, overly warm areas. Sit where there is more likely to be moving air, near a fan or a cracked-open door or window.

5. **Pack it and pull it** – If you have gifts or other items to bring along, tote them in a rolling cart. If you don't have a cart, leave your packages and potluck dish in the car and ask a more able family member to go get them for you. If neither of these is an option, pack your stuff into a backpack or a tote bag, preferably with a long enough strap to go over your head and across your chest. It helps to carry something heavy close to your body, instead of in your hands. This also can keep your hands free to hold on to a railing or the arm of a friend.

6. **Push it** – Use a grocery cart every time you shop, even if you're not buying a lot. Wipe the handle with an anti-bacterial towelette before you grab it. Ask the bagger to pack your bags light. More, lightweight bags are easier to carry than a few heavy ones.

7. **Pump it up** – Although it might be tempting to skip pulmonary rehab class or routine exercise, keep in mind that exercise helps reduce stress and also burns off the extra calories you're likely to consume around this time. Besides that, it's fun to celebrate the holidays with your friends at pulmonary rehab. If you absolutely don't have the time or energy for aerobic exercise, at least do your stretches and strength training. It will keep you feeling good and staying flexible.

8. **Pucker up and Pace** – Use your breathing techniques! You know (or at least I hope you do) that pursed-lips breathing really does make a difference in helping you stay in control of your breathing. Slow down and remind yourself to do it, even if you need to count it out: in one, two…out one, two, three, four. Ahhhh…

9. **Puff your O$_2$** – If your doctor has prescribed supplemental oxygen, wear it. Everybody at that party needs oxygen, for every single breath. You just happen to need a little more. Give your body a break and nourish it with O$_2$. You will be less tired, and your lungs, heart, and brain will be a lot less stressed!

It's Party Time! **Prioritize, Position, Plan, Pace, Pack, Pull, Push, Pump, Pucker, Pace, and Puff. You'll breathe easier and you'll have a great time!**

Your Turn

Key points, or…if you don't remember anything else from this chapter, remember this:

- You can actively participate in holiday events, even if you have COPD.

- The choices you make, even small ones, can mean the difference between having a good time with easy breathing – or a lousy time, struggling for breath.
- You can make good choices – and you must – especially when you are limited by COPD.

Ask yourself this:

How can I remember to use these tips when I attend my next event or party?

This week:

Think of three specific activities (carrying gifts, being overscheduled, etc.) that concern you the most. Review the nine points in this chapter and find one that might help with each issue. Then visualize yourself following the suggestions and breathing better.

Here's more help:

Read or review chapter May – Week 2: Make the Most of the Breath you Have – Energy Conservation and Work Simplification.

December – Week 3

A COPD Christmas

"Never, ever underestimate the importance of having fun."

~ Randy Pausch

A COPD Christmas

Jim Phillips

'Twas the night before Christmas, and all through the house
Not a creature was stirring 'cept me and my spouse.
If you're wondering why, let me do some explaining.
We were doing a thing called bronchial draining.

There I was on my slant board, and she on her knees,
Clapping my chest, while I lie there and wheeze.
When all of a sudden, there arose such a clatter
We ran to the window to see what was the matter.

Imagine our surprise to see out in the yard
An old guy bent over and coughing real hard.
He had a white beard and shiny black boots,
A bag full of gifts and wore a red suit.

As we stared, he stood up, and looking at me,
He said in despair, "I have COPD."
"I've wondered each year when I'm out with my pack
If someone would see when I have an attack."

"I fear that I'm just getting older," said he,
"And soon I'll be on Social Security."
"Come in my dear Santa, and you'll soon be elated,
I'll tell you about being rehabilitated."

"Put yourself in the hands of the team,
Pay close attention and you'll be back on the beam.
The things they will teach will bring you success,
Things like breathing and coughing and handling stress."

"You'll exercise right, with treadmill and weights,
What a change will be seen in your physical state!
You'll eat only good things, watching the pounds,
It'll be a lot easier making your rounds."

"So please, Mr. Santa, give rehab a whirl,
Think of your health for the kids of the world."
He said, "Why you're right, sir, the message is clear,
Rehab's the answer. I'll do it this year!"

And laying a finger aside of his nose,
And pursing his lips, up the chimney he rose.
Using diaphragm breathing, he got on his sleigh,
And with a loud "Merry Christmas!" he went on his way.

Your Turn

Key points, or...if you don't remember anything else from this chapter, remember this:

Sometimes you need to take a break from learning, enjoy yourself, and have fun!

Ask yourself this:

Am I keeping a sense of humor and fun throughout this holiday season?

This week:

Share this poem, or another fun story or poem, with friends, family, and your pals with COPD.

December – Week 4

Thoughts About the Future

"The future is called 'perhaps,' which is the only possible thing to call it. And the important thing is not to allow that to scare you."

~ Tennessee Williams

It's funny, you know...I never really allowed myself to think much about my future after diagnosis. I was, after all, diagnosed with COPD when I was just fifty-two years old. I received the devastating sentence of having this incurable, mostly progressive chronic illness, was told I had between two and five years to live, and had to use supplemental oxygen twenty-four hours a day, seven days a week for the rest of my life.

It took me a long time to work my way through the various stages of acceptance, and to adjust to the lifestyle changes required of me. Some of those adjustments kind of snuck up on me when I wasn't looking and somehow became a part of daily living. Others required commitment and dedication of effort, pulling survival instincts from so deep within me that the intensity still comes as a surprise whenever I think about it.

But survive I did! Even with a grim prognosis, I have somehow come through the obstacle course that God set for me, and now find myself pushing the finish line even further out front.

You see, there is still so much to do! There are sights to be seen, people to help, words to be spoken, and actions to be taken. And try as I might, I can't seem to cram them all into the space of a day – the measure of time we are all given in a twenty-four-hour period – a simple day in which to accomplish all that we set before ourselves.

I guess that's what has led me to begin planning ahead, strangely, for the future. And the future I wouldn't allow myself at first, seems to loom ahead of me now like the proverbial carrot before the nose of a donkey. Take just one more step; do just one more thing; and smell the carrot along the way.

I sometimes startle myself whenever I catch myself thinking about something I want to do a few years down the road. Suddenly I find myself making long-term agreements and signing contracts and leases of several years' duration.

Admittedly, there are times when I prefer to give in to this disease, when I awaken in the morning with a raging headache, or when the fatigue pulls me down as though my feet were mired in molasses. But the whiff of that carrot – my future opportunities to do more, be more, help more – serve to push my feet into action and my brain into gear!

Maintaining stability has allowed me to stay in control of COPD and my overall health. Dr. Tom Petty once said that a disease is an impairment of an organ system, its structure or its function; but an illness is the total impact of that impairment on the life of the person. There is a difference. A person can have COPD, a significant disease – without being constantly sick.

I accept the fact that having COPD limits me, but it makes my heart soar to know it does not change the person I am. Accepting myself as a person with COPD who can still be healthy and enjoy life has given me the peace and the confidence to be able to consider – and see – a future! Carry on, my friends, into the New Year with this knowledge, confidence, and joy.

Your Turn

Key points, or…if you don't remember anything else from this chapter, remember this:

- COPD is not a death sentence.
- With knowledge, determination, and a positive attitude you can look forward to the future.

Ask yourself this:

Do I look at COPD as a loss of lung function, but not the loss of the person I am?

This week:

List three things you are looking forward to in the New Year.

Authors' and Contributors' Biographies

Jane M. Martin, BA, CRT

Jane M. Martin is a respiratory therapist and teacher with over thirty-five years' experience in respiratory care. Working in acute care she became frustrated with the "revolving door" of providing emergency and urgent care to patients with COPD, only to see them return to the hospital not long after with the same problem. Aware that there were over twenty million people in the US with COPD, she was disheartened when time after time she heard patients ask, "Am I the only one who has this problem? What's going to happen to me? How can anybody possibly understand how I feel?"

In response, Jane began developing programs for COPD and asthma, most notably a pulmonary rehabilitation program and chronic lung disease support group. In her work in pulmonary rehabilitation she was inspired by her patients but concerned for others with little or no information and support. She knew that a connection must be made from those people who were lonely, angry, and confused, to those who had learned to live well and thrive in spite of the emotional and physical obstacles found in life with COPD. To this end she wrote *Breathe Better, Live in Wellness: Winning Your Battle Over Shortness of Breath,* sharing stories of everyday people with extraordinary and inspiring wisdom, humor, and courage.

Jane went on to create BreathingBetterLivingWell.com a website providing education and support for people with chronic lung disease, as well as an online community providing information and support for people with COPD and other chronic lung diseases. She is the author of two books on living with COPD and over 100 COPD-related articles.

Originally from the Chicago area, Jane holds a bachelor's degree in education and language arts from Hope College and a degree in respiratory care from the California College for Health Sciences. She works for the COPD Foundation and lives with her husband in West Michigan.

Jo-Von Tucker

At age fifty-two Jo-Von Tucker was told she had COPD, that she would need to wear oxygen twenty-four-hours a day for the rest of her life, and that she had two to five years to live. Determined to beat the odds, she set out to learn all she could about COPD but found very little. As a result, she made it her mission to do all she could to provide information and support to people with COPD and their families.

Prior to her diagnosis of COPD, Jo-Von owned a successful direct marketing consulting firm specializing in upscale catalogs. In the course of her career she received more than 400 national and international design, writing, and marketing awards. She traveled extensively, speaking and consulting to those in the direct marketing industry.

After diagnosis she moved to Cape Cod, Massachusetts, and acquired Clambake Celebrations, a company specializing in marketing and shipping live, fresh lobster and clambake feasts throughout the United States. Not long after this, Clambake Celebrations was selected as one of the Top 100 Small Business Websites in America by Small Business Computing Magazine.

Jo-Von was the author of *Courage and Information for Life with COPD*, a groundbreaking work combining scientific and medical information about COPD with a patient's unique insights. As founder and leader of the Cape Cod COPD Support Group she created a sense of sharing and community for people with COPD. Her newsletters, distributed to patients and healthcare professionals throughout the country, contained news of current events in the world of COPD, locally and nationally.

Jo-Von was born in Dallas, Texas, and lived and worked in New York for many years before moving to Cape Cod. She attended the University of Texas in Austin. Fourteen years after her initial diagnosis of COPD Jo-Von passed away unexpectedly from complications following surgery. For more about Jo-Von Tucker, see A Story of Two Women at the beginning of this book.

Contributor Biographies

Francis V. Adams, MD

Francis V. Adams is a New York City pulmonologist in private practice. Dr. Adams received his BA from Georgetown University and medical degree from Cornell Medical College. He is an associate professor of clinical medicine at New York University and an attending physician at the NYU Langone Medical Center and Bellevue Hospital in New York.

In 2006 Dr. Adams was sworn in as a police surgeon for the NYPD. He is the author of *The Asthma Sourcebook*, *The Breathing Disorders Sourcebook*, and *Healing Through Empathy,* among other works. Dr. Adams is a contributor to *The LA Times* and hosts *Doctor*

Radio on SiriusXM 110 weekly. He has been named as one of the best doctors in the city by *New York Magazine* and in *Top Doctors: New York Metro Area* by Castle Connolly Medical Ltd.

Dr. Adams has been interviewed on television, radio, and the Internet regarding his books and quoted on the subject of asthma in newspaper and magazine articles. He has maintained a web site (www.adamsmd.com) for several years, which includes a news page listing the current advances in lung disease. Dr. Adams publishes an electronic newsletter weekly which is obtainable through his web site.

Robert A. Sandhaus, MD, PhD, FCCP

Dr. Robert Sandhaus has fifty years of experience in medicine and research aimed at improving our understanding of alpha1-antitrypsin deficiency and related disorders. He is board-certified in the specialty areas of internal medicine, pulmonary disease, and critical care medicine.

He is a founding member of the Boards of AlphaNet, the Alpha-1 Foundation, and the Alpha-1 Project. Since 2000 he has held the position of Medical Director of AlphaNet and AlphaNet Canada, and Clinical Director of the Alpha-1 Foundation. Dr. Sandhaus also serves as a faculty member at the National Jewish Health in Denver, where he is professor of medicine and has directed the Alpha-1 Program for nearly forty years.

Dr. Sandhaus received a BA in Molecular Biology from Haverford College and went on to receive a PhD in experimental pathology and a medical degree at the Stony Brook University. He has held academic positions at Harvard Medical School, the University of California at San Francisco, and the University of Colorado. Dr. Sandhaus was born in Cleveland, Ohio; and currently lives in Bow Mar, Colorado, with his family.

Vijai Sharma, PhD

Vijai Sharma, PhD, is a retired clinical psychologist who endured untreated asthma and chronic bronchitis since childhood and was not diagnosed with emphysema until 1994. Dr. Sharma specialized in mind-body medicine early in his professional practice, understanding that anxiety, depression, anger, pain, and stress can affect cardiopulmonary, digestive, and immune system functions. He believes that we can utilize the body, breath, mind, and spiritual energy for personal well-being, overall health, and a better quality of life.

Dr. Sharma received extensive clinical training in India, the United Kingdom, and Sweden, and in 1981, was licensed as a clinical psychologist in Tennessee. He completed advanced teachers' training in yoga and believes that yoga has helped him psychologically and physically in his battle with emphysema. Today he strictly follows recommended COPD medical treatment along with a program of wide-ranging exercise, yoga, nutrition, and self-care focusing especially on meditation, mindfulness, and walking.

Helen M. Sorenson MA, RRT, CPFT, FAARC

Helen M. Sorenson is a retired registered respiratory therapist, and former associate professor in the Department of Respiratory Care at the University of Texas Health Science Center in San Antonio, Texas. She received a degree in biology from Dana College in Blair, Nebraska; a certificate of completion from California College for Respiratory Care and earned the CRT, CPFT and RRT credentials from the National Board for Respiratory Care.

In 2000 she was awarded a Master of Arts (MA) degree in social gerontology from the University of Nebraska in Omaha. In 2014 she was awarded The Practitioner of the Year Award, Education Specialty Section from the American Association for Respiratory Care

(AARC). She recently updated a chapter on geriatrics for the textbook, Respiratory Care Principles and Practices, 4th Edition 2020, and continues to write articles for the AARC Times when requested.

In addition to the joy of her three children and five grandchildren she enjoys reading, crocheting, and traveling with her husband, and remains active in her church.

Glossary

Acute: An illness that comes on suddenly and lasts a few hours or days.

Airway obstruction: A blocking or narrowing of the airways on their way to or within the lung.

Allergen: A substance causing inflammation in the lungs. Common allergens are pollen, animal dander, dust mites, and mold.

Alpha-1 Antitrypsin Deficiency: A genetically inherited condition in which the liver does not make enough of a protein that protects the lungs and liver from damage, leading to emphysema and liver disease. Patients with Alpha-1 Antitrypsin Deficiency develop severe emphysema in their 20's, 30's, and 40's.

Alveoli: Tiny sac-like structures at the ends of the airways where the exchange of oxygen and carbon dioxide takes place.

Antibiotic: A drug that kills or inhibits bacteria.

Apnea: The absence of breathing, usually longer than ten seconds. Obstructive sleep apnea is a condition in which breathing stops during sleep due to an obstruction in the airway. Central sleep apnea is a condition in which, for some reason, the respiratory center in the brain fails to send the message to breathe.

Arterial blood gas (ABG): A blood test drawn from the artery to determine how well the lungs are working relative to other metabolic functions of the body.

Asthma: An obstructive lung disease characterized by airway hyper-responsiveness, inflammation, narrowing, and spasm.

Asthmatic bronchitis: A type of bronchitis commonly associated with COPD involving cough, airway hyper-responsiveness, and mucus production.

Bacteria: Infectious organisms that may produce bronchitis or pneumonia as well as illness elsewhere in the body.

BiPAP (Bi-level Positive Airway Pressure – inspiratory and expiratory): A mechanical device used to assist breathing in severe lung disease, following surgery, or in obstructive sleep apnea. This treatment is "non-invasive," meaning that no tube is inserted into the lungs. Pressure is applied to the respiratory airways via a mask that can be quite easily and quickly put on and removed.

Biomarker: A defined characteristic that is measured as an indicator of normal biological processes, pathogenic processes, or responses to an exposure or intervention, including therapeutic interventions.

Bleb: Destroyed, non-functional part of the lung that takes up space and puts pressure on a less damaged portion of the lung.

Bronchial hygiene: Keeping the lungs free of excess mucus by using inhalers, nebulizer treatments, percussion and postural drainage, systemic hydration, effective cough techniques, or mechanical devices that aid in airway clearance.

Bronchitis: Irritation of the lining of the bronchial airways, characterized by a frequent cough.

Bronchiectasis: Chronic infection often found in the lower parts of the lung, characterized by copious amounts of excess mucus and dilated bronchial airways.

Bronchus: The two main divisions from the trachea, each one leading into a lung. There are approximately twenty additional sets of branches before reaching the alveoli.

Cannula: A soft plastic device used to deliver oxygen. Worn on the face and held in place by the ears, it has two short prongs positioned in the nares (nostrils).

Capillaries: Tiny blood vessels surrounding the alveoli. Oxygen and carbon dioxide pass through the walls of the capillaries to get into and out of the lungs.

Carbon Dioxide (CO_2): The waste product of respiration that is removed from the body through exhalation.

Chronic: Disease that has been present for a longer period of time, usually months or years.

Cilia: Tiny hair like structures that line the bronchial airways and sweep mucus upward toward the mouth. Cilia cleanse the lungs and defend against irritants and can be destroyed by cigarette smoke and pollution.

Cor Pulmonale: Strain of the right side of the heart due to chronic lung disease.

CPAP (Continuous Positive Airway Pressure - inspiratory): A mechanical device used to assist breathing and in the treatment of obstructive sleep apnea. This treatment is "non-invasive," meaning no tube is inserted into the lungs. Pressure is applied to the respiratory airways by way of a mask that is quite easily and quickly put on and removed.

Diaphragm: The main muscle of breathing. The diaphragm is a large sheet of muscle separating the chest and the abdomen.

Diaphragmatic breathing: A method of breathing in which the diaphragm is used to a greater extent than are the accessory breathing muscles.

Dyspnea: Difficulty breathing, shortness of breath.

Emphysema: Destruction or enlargement of the alveoli; a condition in which the alveoli lose their elasticity and become stretched out and floppy.

Exacerbation: An episodic worsening of a chronic illness.

FEV_1: Forced expiratory volume in the first second of exhalation in a pulmonary function test. This number is helpful in determining the degree of airway obstruction.

Holding chamber: A handheld device, usually plastic, containing a one-way valve, used with a metered dose inhaler (MDI), assisting in maximum delivery of medication to the lungs.

Inflammation: Irritated, reddened, and swollen tissue.

Irritants: Substances that irritate the airways, causing swelling and increased mucus production. Common irritants are smoke, smog, aerosol sprays, and perfume.

Metabolism: The consumption of nutrients combined with oxygen, which produces energy and maintains living tissue.

Nebulizer: A breathing treatment in which liquid medication becomes a fine mist to be inhaled into the lungs. Can be taken in a medical facility or at home.

Non-invasive: A medical test or procedure that is done with no tubes, needles, or other devices going through the skin or otherwise into the body. For example: an electrocardiogram or an ultrasound of the heart is non-invasive. A bronchoscopy, with a tube and tiny camera going into the lungs, is considered as invasive.

NTM lung disease: Nontuberculous mycobacterial lung disease is a serious infection caused by a type of NTM bacteria. When it gets into the lungs, NTM bacteria can invade the cells that protect the lungs from infection. This can lead to chronic lung infections and pneumonia.

Obstructive sleep apnea (OSA): A blockage of the airway causing the absence of breathing during sleep, sometimes hundreds of times during the night and often for a minute or longer.

Oxygen: (O$_2$): A gas needed to sustain human life. Earth's atmosphere is 20.9% oxygen.

Oxygen saturation (O$_2$ Sat): A measure of oxygen saturation in the blood, measured in percent and often obtained with a pulse oximeter.

Pneumonia: A common infection in people with COPD caused by bacteria or virus.

Pneumothorax: Lung collapse causing air to leak from within the lung into the space between the lung and the chest wall, causing pain and difficulty breathing.

Pulmonary function test: A medical test resulting in measurements of air movement – speed, volume, and flow – as well as diffusion of oxygen. Can be done in a complete or abbreviated form, depending upon information required by the physician.

Pulse oximeter: A device used to determine the percent of oxygen saturation in the blood. This test is quick, easy, non-invasive, and painless.

Pursed-lips breathing: A method of breathing which prolongs the expiratory phase, increasing the amount of carbon dioxide expelled; it slows down breathing and allows the person using this method to increase control over breathing.

Respirator: See "ventilator."

Respiratory failure: A chronic or acute state in which the lungs are unable to provide enough oxygen to the body and/or remove enough carbon dioxide from the body.

Sleep study: A study done to observe various physiologic changes during sleep. Done overnight, in a laboratory.

SOB: Short of Breath, or Shortness of Breath

Spacer: A handheld device, usually plastic, used with metered dose inhaler (MDI) to assist with increased delivery of medication to the lungs.

Spirometer: A device used to measure lung function. This is different from an "incentive spirometer" used to encourage deep breathing exercise, often used after surgery.

Spirometry: A lung function test measuring the volume and speed of air being inhaled and exhaled.

Supplemental oxygen: A term used to describe oxygen therapy, oxygen taken into the body from a mechanical or pressurized source other than room air.

Trachea: The main airway leading to both lungs. Sometimes referred to as the windpipe.

Transtracheal catheter: A small tube inserted into a hole in the trachea supplying oxygen to the lungs. Used for long-term supplemental oxygen consumption in which a higher flow is required and/or if the patient does not wish to have a nasal cannula visible.

Ventilator: A mechanical device used to treat respiratory failure or provide respiratory support following surgery. Tubing from the ventilator is connected to an endotracheal tube inserted into the patient's lungs via the mouth or nose. Also referred to as a respirator.

Virus: A group of highly contagious infectious agents causing head colds and chest infections as well as illness elsewhere in the body. Antibiotics are ineffective against viruses. Vaccination against the influenza virus (flu shot) is effective.

Wheeze: A whistling sound of air entering or leaving the lungs, commonly found in asthma.

Resources

COPD Foundation
http://www.copdfoundation.org
866-731-2673

Learn More, Breathe Better Program
http://www.nhlbi.nih.gov/health/public/lung/copd/lmbb-campaign/index.htm
877-645-2448

National Jewish Health
http://www.nationaljewish.org
800-222-5864

The Pulmonary Paper
http://www.pulmonarypaper.org
800-950-3698

Sea Puffers – Pulmonary Cruises
http://www.seapuffers.com
866-673-3019

Well Spouse Association / Family Caregiver Alliance
http://www.wellspouse
900-838-0879